THE SECRET OF
THE GOLDEN PHALLUS
MALE EROTIC ALCHEMY FOR THE 21ST CENTURY

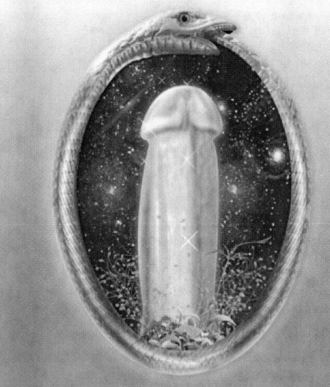

BRUCE P. GRETHER

LETHE PRESS
MAPLE SHADE NJ

Book Design by Toby Johnson
Artwork and drawings by Bruce P. Grether

Published as a trade paperback original
by Lethe Press, 118 Heritage Avenue, Maple Shade, NJ 08052.
April, 2012
ISBN 1-59021-118-9   ISBN-13 978-1-59021-118-2

Library of Congress Cataloging-in-Publication Data

Grether, Bruce P., 1953-
 The secret of the golden phallus : male erotic alchemy for the 21st century / Bruce P. Grether.
    p. cm.
Includes bibliographical references.
ISBN-13: 978-1-59021-118-2
ISBN-10: 1-59021-118-9
1. Masturbation. 2. Penis--Erection. 3. Sexual excitement. I. Title.
HQ447.G74 2012
306.77'2--dc23
                                                2012008441

This one is for Tom, forever;
our beloved Brother N.M., for always;
and Nils, a NextGen Wiseman.

Contents

The Magick Power of Your Self-Pleasure
Three Forms of Male Solosex Magick
A Mindful Masturbation Mantra
Churning the Ocean of Milk
How to Take a New Erotic Imprint
Golden Phallus Yoga
You Are the New Adam of the New Earth

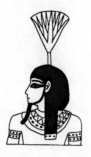

THE SECRET OF THE GOLDEN PHALLUS

*Had I not observed that Purblinde men have discoursed well of sight,
and some without issue, excellently of Generation; I that was never master
of any considerable garden, had not attempted on this subject. But the
Earth is the Garden of Nature, and each fruitfull Country a Paradise...*

— Sir Thomas Browne
The Garden of Cyrus, 1658

*The tendency of Nature is in the direction of the dominant activity of
the Positive pole.*

—Three Initiates
The Kybalion: Hermetic Philosophy, 1912, p. 156

I have masturbated myself out of serious problems in my life.

— John Mayer
Rolling Stone Magazine, Feb., 2010

INTRODUCTION

BY JOSEPH KRAMER, PhD
IN HUMAN SEXUALITY

Why do boys and men joke about masturbation? Why are we embarrassed to speak of "pure penile pleasure"? Is masturbation a poor substitution for the real thing? Is masturbation shameful, dirty, sinful and vulgar? Is sex with our selves too intimate to speak about? Or is masturbation at the core of who we are?

Bruce P. Grether has spent most of the last fifteen years as a male masturbation activist and teacher. We first became friends in the mid nineties. He wrote to me that thanks to my video *Fire on the Mountain—Male Genital Massage,* he took something he loved doing anyway—masturbating—and turned it into a profound practice that helped him access expanded erotic states. Now that he understood the power of prolonged sexual arousal, he said he understood many ancient myths differently, especially the story of the Egyptian fertility god Min.

Bruce has evolved into a missionary for male masturbation as a practice to enhance self-esteem, stimulate personal growth, heal and even transform one's self. Online, in DVDs, and in classes, Bruce teaches that the sustained sexual arousal produced from Mindful Masturbation gives us access to the magic deep within our hearts. This is the message of *The Secret of the Golden Phallus.* We have the power. Do not be afraid. Our aroused body is where it happens.

Towards the end of *The Secret of the Golden Phallus,* Bruce calls on us to practice Golden Phallus Yoga, which has "no precise description or set of instructions." He says this yoga manifests when we simply listen to the innate wisdom of our own bodies. Much of this book was "written" while Bruce was in high erotic states. It is most appropriate for the reader of this text to also be aroused.

Enjoy your Golden Phallus.

PREFACE

This book is about only one thing: your relationship with your penis. Your sexual identity is not the primary issue here, rather this book is aimed at *all* human males, regardless of how you may label your sexuality. Your penis is a key factor and yet in order to benefit from the secrets revealed, you must invite your entire body to participate in your erotic enjoyment. You need to view all of your parts as a greater whole.

That miraculous male organ rooted between your legs has been trivialized and demonized for centuries by human authorities—because when you really surrender to the phallic energy, the experience is extremely empowering, liberating and sacred. Then you need no external authority; you need no intermediary with the Divine; you know that you have everything you need.

In this book the term "Divine" is not meant in a religious sense, rather it refers to whatever larger picture includes you and everything that exists—which you may prefer to call the Universe, the Source, or even Nature.

The ancestral design of your human male body, along with the inherent phallic wisdom recorded in your many trillions of cells, is your sacred path to connect with your origins as a Son of Gaia, the Earth.

This experience and awareness is subversive indeed!

To totally turn around all the weird and destructive attitudes towards the penis, and shift the energy invested there instead to honor and celebrate your precious male genitalia, can not only transform you—it also contributes to creating a better world for everyone.

The subject of this book is not theoretical; it is experiential.

Likewise, though you will find plenty of vivid stories and symbols of phallic mythology, none of the images are actually abstract or separate from the direct experience of your own body that brings them to life. Every story here in reality is about *you*, your male body, your penis, and its erection. Your genitals are the flowering of your human body, and that bloom provides your sacred seed. Your genitals are to be honored and admired just as you honor and admire flowers in a garden.

Among the mistaken, acquired beliefs many men still suffer is that your actual human penis is too ordinary and mundane to be called a "phallus," much less to be considered divine. As you break those cultural agreements—which you did not make, but were made for you by others—you can seize your own divine nature as a vibrant part of the greater picture of Nature itself. Do this at the same time that you literally take hold of yourself and grasp your personal power.

Here are truths about your male sexual nature and erotic energy that have been hidden from you by cultural conditioning. Most of what you have been taught to believe about human sexuality, your male body, and your penis is simply not true.

This book will reawaken from within you things you already know, yet may have forgotten, or even pushed aside from direct awareness. It is time to look at these things directly again and to bring them out into the light of day. For example: penile erection is your direct connection with your own divinity and makes it tangible, actual, and undeniable. Pure penile pleasure is a direct connection with the Divine.

Arousal and erotic ecstasy awakens phallic wisdom within your cells. All of your male ancestors stir in the DNA matrix of your body with the stimulation of your erection.

Most of these men probably never had the opportunity to experience the kind of high-quality abundant erotic bliss that is now available to you as their heir, their latest embodied expression.

The phallic energy is extremely powerful: creative, sustaining, and regenerative.

When fully activated, this energy brings back together into wholeness all that may have seemed separated or fragmented within you. It also regenerates your connection with other people and the world you live in. Your penis is the living image of that World Axis that connects the Above and the Below, that merges all dualistic polarities, and manifests the dynamic flow of creative energy—the same mysterious energy that creates the world.

As you recognize this energy in your own body, you align your being with the way the world is organized. You *are* the microcosm of the macrocosm.

To reclaim this connection aligns you with the creative processes of Creation itself.

Total, unadulterated adoration for your penis offers empowerment and autonomy unavailable anywhere else. To love your penis and the ecstasy that it provides, without reservation, is to claim your inheritance as a phallic god. As such, a god is simply the personification of a universal force. Such a god is a powerful potential within you, a divine spark that may remain dormant or merely potential until you invite it to unfold into full expression.

Your sacred phallus *is* the Tree of Life whose leaves are for the healing of the nations, whose flowering is your limitless bliss, and whose fruit is the phallic god within you that emerges into manifestation when you practice Male Erotic Alchemy.

Everyone is conditioned to some extent with limiting beliefs about the male body and genitals.

Consider this: *Why do the erect penis and male masturbation remain far stronger taboos overall on this planet, than even the taboo against male homosexual behavior?*

In the present day, mainstream media and films often portray homosexuality in quite sympathetic terms. Not so with explicit erections and male masturbation, except to trivialize or demonize them by implication. Such depictions remain the province of farcical jokes, condemnation, furtive secrecy, or are relegated to the multi-billion dollar per year porn industry.

As of this writing, in mainstream films no one displays a full erection, and you will definitely *not* see a man actually masturbating.

This tells you something crucial!

As you absorb what this book tells you, everything you see in the world makes more sense—the world speaks to you, as you learn to listen with your whole being.

Likewise, what you see anchored between your legs takes on deeper and higher significance than you ever imagined. There are no limits to where it can take you.

In the chapters that follow you are introduced to what many millions of people consider the most sacred mountain in the world, a phallic image over 27,000 feet high. You will explore the most ancient phallic myths and learn how these are directly relevant to you here and now in your own body. You will learn exactly how to practice Male Erotic Alchemy, which is the process of personal transformation and regeneration through states of high erotic ecstasy. Only by going on the full journey can you circle back to reclaim your deepest essential self.

This book offers you guidance through a progressive practice of phallic self-discovery and transformation:

- **Mindful Masturbation**
- **Male Erotic Alchemy**
- **Golden Phallus Yoga**

With Male Erotic Alchemy you will find an emphasis upon male self-pleasure as a spiritual practice. **Mindful Masturbation is a key practice involved in Male Erotic Alchemy, along with the Three Varieties of Male Solosex Magick, and Erotic Re-Imprinting, all of which lead you to Golden Phallus Yoga.** One important reason for this solosexual emphasis is that with self-pleasure you can avoid the dependency and distractions that may arise in partnered sex as you explore your erotic potential using Mindful Masturbation. In solosexual practice you can keep the focus effectively upon developing your skills and erotic fitness.

No major religion now affirms the phallus as a sacred image, or gives approval to the Male Mysteries. Though the Shiva-lingam is honored as a symbol in Hinduism, many Hindus now deny its literal phallic associations, partly due to a certain Victorian prudishness acquired during British rule. Indeed the direct experience of the Male Mysteries is often condemned and reviled precisely because it is so powerful and empowering to you as an embodied human male. With an open mind and heart and passionate belief in yourself, you can reclaim this natural heritage from its current obscurity.

There is a certain amount of truth to the saying that "Some things never change," or at least some things truly have a timeless quality. This is why the stories of the ancient Egyptian phallic gods and their parallel, related phallic deities—the similitude of Osiris and Shiva—are relevant to you today. The essence of the phallic significance of both gods has not changed and is key to the Secret of the Golden Phallus.

This book tells you how to listen deeply to your penis for the purpose of exploring beyond all previous limitations of your erotic experience.

At the same time, Male Erotic Alchemy as you learn it here is designed to be totally user-friendly. You may even skip to chapters seven-through-ten which contain the core of specific instructions for actual practice. Chapter Ten by itself contains the most essential instructions. However, to most fully benefit overall, you may wish to return later to the archetypal tales, which will deepen the rewards of your practice as they trigger cellular memories below the conscious level.

Your amazing penis has an ancient and honorable history and a legacy of mythic, legendary, religious and spiritual significance that illuminates and can inspire you as an embodied, highly sexual human male, if you embrace the images and the literal realities they point to in your own incredible human body and erotic experience.

The mythic imagery is important and extremely powerful because it speaks directly to your unconscious mind. Though you may consciously follow the narrative, the imagery of what happens and what you *see* in these stories speaks below the verbal level to your entire body/mind system. By a computer analogy, your conscious mind is like the display on your monitor; the major operating system is the unconscious mind, comprised of all the rest, including both software and hardware. This analogy even extends to your Internet and wireless connections with the Global Brain, which you can call the *collective unconscious*.

You may notice that the spiritual impulse here is not that of transcendence, rather, it is immanence. Transcendence often involves escapism or avoidance of the physical, material reality; immanence views the Divine as expressed everywhere, in everything, here and now. You are encouraged to be present and embodied.

I am grateful to Joseph Kramer, whose remarkable teaching of Taoist Erotic Massage led me to create my practice of Mindful Masturbation. The Body Electric School, which he created, is an excellent introduction to conscious erotic practice. I am likewise grateful to Toby Johnson, whose writings on gay spirituality and whose deep understanding of erotic energy are great inspirations.

Pause often as you read this material. Close the book, spread your thighs wide and reach between your legs for the Secret of the Golden Phallus that already belongs to you. Everything you really need is there in the wisdom of your cells. However, most men do need the kind of reminders contained in this book to re-awaken this inner knowing. Your pure penile pleasure summons this awareness from within you just as a beautiful garden grows with loving irrigation from its unseen roots into the warm sunshine.

Read the paragraph above again; this time read it *aloud to yourself*—then look between your legs.

Smile!

Chapter One:

Your Male Ancestors Live within You

When you look down along your torso, at the base of your belly, rooted between your thighs is a most amazing and powerful organ. You have probably been told many times that your complex and highly evolved brain is your most important organ. You may hear that your brain is actually "where it all happens," however, deep within you, you know that is only part of the truth.

Without the direct participation of your penis to generate the actual sensations, your brain can only indulge in fantasy about things that are not really happening.

Almost every man on the planet has a natural obsession with his penis. Plus, understandably every man is naturally drawn to the extraordinary sensations his penis can generate for him. In fact, your attitude toward your penis is at the core of your attitude toward yourself and how you feel about your entire life.

Less fortunate is the fact that this relationship is not always free of guilt, shame, fear and superstition. Most men do have some mixed feelings about their body and penis, due to a combination of conditioning and personal history.

Aside from such acquired ambivalence—which is something worth working on—if you are honest with yourself, your penis stands at the center of your identity as a male human being. This is perfect and right. It is absolutely as it ought to be.

Any mixed feelings only obscure the truth and goodness of this identification.

It is also natural and healthy, that if you find your own penis fascinating and wonderful, you are interested in the penises of your fellow men. Most men have some such curiosity and interest, and always have. The manner in which men in public restrooms tend to sneak a look at the fellow urinating beside them indicates this. It has nothing much to do with what we now label "sexual orientation" or "preference."

It's more of a human male fascination, as the penis is physically so obvious, being an external organ that can radically change size, that waxes and wanes from rigid and hot to extremely soft and delicately cooler; on every level its significance is intense and profound. Most men have an innate interest in penises, erections, and male bodies in general, regardless of so-called sexuality—for that is what every man sees when he looks at his own body.

Your attitude toward your penis is equivalent to your attitude toward yourself.

That is the plain truth.

Your amazing penis is the current incarnation of thousands of human ancestors, and millions of male ancestors from before humans existed. These male ancestors all remain recorded and alive in essence within the cells and molecules of your body.

With every living pulse of your arousal, with each tingle of penile stimulation, those male ancestors within you enjoy and celebrate *your* ecstatic sensations.

You are all of them; they are always part of you.

The Most Sacred Mountain in the World

The great rounded head of dark stone thrusts upward against a sky deepened to blue-violet by the extremely high altitude among snow-laden peaks. Amid spectacular yet severe surroundings, the rising horizontal strata of rock that support this particular domed head stand in the midst of an immense geological trough all around its base. The summit of this astonishing peak looks like an almost-perfect natural pyramid. In one of the most remote and inhospitable corners of the world stands this remarkable peak, the sacred mountain called Kailash.

It rises 21,778 feet above sea level at the far western edge of Tibet. The extremely vertical mass of Kailash climbs in a series of dramatic striations. It is considered to actually *be* Shiva-lingam incarnate—the erect penis of the ancient Indus Valley Lord of Animals, Horned God, Lord of Yogis, Lord of the Dance: the Regenerator, a god later known as Lord Shiva.

Kailash is considered so sacred that no one is allowed to climb to the summit.

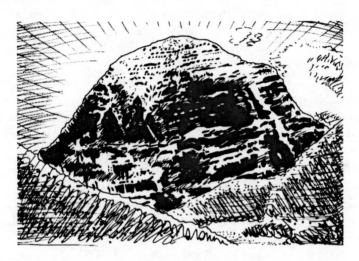

Mount Kailash

In fact, the peak is sacred to three major modern religions: Hinduism, followers of ancient Tibetan Bön, and also Buddhism. Though no one is allowed to climb it, in recent years the annual pilgrimage has resumed, an arduous journey to venerate the sacred mountain and trek around it. To make the thirty-two mile hike required in order to circle the foot of Mount Kailash is said to bestow a great blessing.

Most traditional belief systems on the planet include a mountain considered supremely sacred, as the "home of the gods," the axis of the world, the navel of the Universe, or a peak upon which someone is said to have encountered the Divine. Because of its ancient and unusual history, however, Kailash may be said to be the most sacred summit of all. This veneration predates any surviving modern religion. No doubt the mountain itself was worshiped as a Holy Lingam long before its god was personified.

Just as Shiva originates with the ancient Indus Valley culture, veneration for Kailash goes back some 5000 years or more. The roots of Yoga are believed to go back at least that far or even longer, and Shiva—whose name means "the Auspicious One"—is credited with being the first Yogi. He remains in essence, the exemplary Yogi for modern practitioners of Yoga.

Tradition tells that from Kailash originate the four great rivers that divide the world into four quarters; this turns out to be quite close to the literal truth for that part of the world. To this day, four of the greatest rivers of South Asia originate near the foot of Kailash: the Indus, the Sutlej, the Brahamaputra, and the Karnali, which is a tributary of the mighty and highly revered Ganges River.

The people of the Indus Valley culture must have known well this remarkable geological phallic image—the mighty shaft of naked rock still said to be the home of Shiva today. The Lord of Yogis is described as sitting naked and cross-legged upon the summit of Kailash in perpetual meditation. He also sports a perpetual erection called the Shiva-lingam, which is literally the World Axis. It connects Below with Above.

This Mountain God has three eyes, with his Third Eye vertical on the middle of his brow. As the Below and Above reflect one another, you can imagine how the two horizontal eyes echo his testicles, while the vertical eye above them parallels his erect phallus.

From the summit of Kailash his presence anchors the continuation of the world through its constant, ongoing cycle of creation, sustaining, and regeneration.

The Indus Valley people credited the God of the Mountain and the Mountain of the God with provision of the flowing waters that brought them fertile soil from upstream with the annual monsoon floods, as well as irrigating their crops through the rest of the year. As such, the Mountain God was Lord of Animals, Pillar of the Sky, the Supreme Deity. The Male Trinity of the Triple God: Creator, Sustainer, and Regenerator.

For them, this awesome deity was no abstract symbol or idea, any more than your penis is merely a thought, or that your penis represents something else. Your penis can represent itself and that's significant enough.

The Mountain God was a living, vibrant and sacred reality to the ancients of the Indus Valley, just as your human penis, its erection and its blissful sensations of pure penile pleasure that nourish your soul are real for you in your daily life.

Ask your penis about this: deep in your cells your body remembers exactly why Mount Kailash remains today a most sacred mountain.

The male ancestors within you know this for the literal truth it is.

What is Male Erotic Alchemy?

A lchemy is an ancient philosophy and practice to transform mundane or common existence into the truly precious, the rare, and the extraordinary. In some versions of alchemy, this is described as the quest for the "Philosopher's Stone," a potent essence that can change base metals into silver or gold. Alchemists also seek to produce an elixir of long life, or immortality, and to learn the perennial wisdom.

During the last five hundred years alchemy has come to be viewed as an arcane, obscure metaphysical study, or a philosophical indulgence that involves vivid symbols and mythic archetypes. However, the evolution of traditional alchemy during the same period led to our current chemistry and physics, and has even contributed to the biology and philosophical thinking of today.

Yet a more timeless, *actual* core of alchemy that you can practice exists.

In reality, alchemy has always been about the inner awareness and transformative potential of the alchemist to connect and unite with the Divine.

This is the quest for your own divine essence, through practices that expand awareness and refine consciousness. In a sense it returns you to where you have always been, only without those conditioned beliefs about who and what you are, beliefs that you no longer need as you continue to evolve. Indeed, those acquired beliefs and agreements become a hindrance on your path and must be discarded. When you drop resistance to what IS, your sense of separation collapses; you feel your Oneness with All Things.

Male Erotic Alchemy refines you to your essence as a natural animal, a living embodied being that is part of the Living Universe. You realize that everything is alive; everything is sacred. You accomplish this shift of awareness when you merge the apparent dualities of matter and spirit, body and mind, or minus (–) and plus (+) charges. Such polarities return to their actual Oneness.

Duality exists only as a way to regard integral, dynamic processes, such as the observation that a full day consists of daytime and nighttime; yet those two work together within a greater whole cycle. Duality is not necessarily bad, only to take it too seriously can be limiting and even destructive. For example, day and night are wonderful, necessary contrasts in your daily cycle of living; they are not actually separate and conflicting opposites.

Taken too far, separation and opposition are the root cause of all suffering.

For human males, the most effective and natural means to accomplish the return to essential Oneness is simply to explore the deeper and higher potentials of the body, the penis, and erotic energy, and by the practice of Male Erotic Alchemy.

This is something your male human body is exquisitely designed for.

Mindful Masturbation is the first step toward the practice of Male Erotic Alchemy. **To masturbate mindfully means *you consciously and deliberately break acquired habits of masturbatory and sexual behavior in order to retrain yourself for optimal self-pleasure, you re-engineer your experience of erotic energy, and you learn to pay full attention to your own body and your sensations while you masturbate.*** To accomplish this you must develop erotic fitness by regular practice, and continuously refine your skills at generating high states of ecstasy. Personal growth, increased self-esteem and self-love, which lead to conscious evolution—this is the actual goal of alchemy.

Mindful Masturbation *provides universally human, science-based insight that helps the body/mind fusion optimize both hormones and brain chemistry to enhance health and happiness and expand consciousness.* Mindful Masturbation works *with* natural body function in a way that helps to counteract the toxic effects of stress.

Mindful Masturbation generates increased nervous system signals that travel both ways between genitals and brain.

This naturally, gradually, and safely opens your heart.

As a water-lily opens to the morning sun…

What is called Serpent Power rising along the spine in Yoga, plus the opening of the seven chakras, or energy centers situated in ascending order through the torso from root to crown, can be accomplished most safely and easily via Mindful Masturbation. It happens naturally and effectively for men through surrender to what the body is designed for, which is to enjoyably, ecstatically achieve balance and happiness on all levels.

A true ecstatic is not a person who only wants to feel pleasure, or wants to feel good all the time. That would be unbalanced, even if it were possible, which it may not be for humans. It is tempting and easy to retreat from suffering into hedonistic escapism, or into a benumbed lack of feeling, hence to sleepwalk in avoidance of pain through the rest of your life. Either way you will probably live as a chronic victim.

However, that is not really living.

A true ecstatic is a person genuinely alive to the entire spectrum of embodied existence; this is not mere self-indulgence, no, it requires courage and persistence. Of course, to live as an ecstatic brings you richer enjoyment than any other way to live.

Still, it is not just about feeling good.

Ecstasy is surrender to the flow of feeling totally alive, fearlessly open to the full range of human experience, from the deepest suffering to the highest exaltation. As an ecstatic you must surrender resistance to what IS. Understandably humans often resist unpleasant experience, however when you simply allow everything to be as it IS, a great deal of energy returns to you that you had invested in resistance to what you disliked. It takes a lot more energy to stay unhappy, than it does to be happy, which in a strong contrast actually generates energy!

When you learn to generate increasing amounts of ecstasy this helps you to maintain balance in your life, for human existence inevitably includes some pain and sadness as well.

The practice called Mindful Masturbation, diligently pursued, can provide all of the core benefits traditionally ascribed to the arcane practices of Taoist cultivation, Serpent Power Yoga, and Tantra. The essence of how those processes work in the body/mind continuum is now well enough understood that the veils of occult secrecy can be lifted. Mindful Masturbation is the entry point for Male Erotic Alchemy, in which you will learn the Three Modes of Male Solosex Magick.

Then you may become an Erotic Wizard who practices Golden Phallus Yoga and apply this to all of your sexual experiences.

These processes are essentially simple, and incredibly powerful, yet they also require that you pay full attention, that you open your mind and heart to break old acquired habits, in order to retrain yourself in the basics. This does not happen in five minutes, or even a year; rather, to fully enact it, this process requires dedicated practice for the remainder of your lifetime.

It will also bring you far greater pleasure than you have ever experienced before.

Amazingly enough, once you grasp the beneficial power of conscious abdominal breathing, deliberate relaxation, plus creative variety and experimentation while you pleasure yourself, your enjoyment of pure penile pleasure will continually increase—it only gets better and better.

The possibilities are truly limitless, as your own experience can demonstrate.

Just as the fingers of a musician or painter, or the vocal cords of a singer continue to learn and develop natural talent with ongoing creative use, your penis actually *learns* to provide you with ever better and finer sensations. You literally train your penis and it learns; it develops new networks of ever-increasing nerve-fiber sensitivity and enhances its connections with all the rest of your body and your brain. At the same time your brain continues to develop pathways to explore ever-finer erotic bliss.

This re-wiring and re-creation is not likely to happen when you masturbate or engage in sexual activity in a habitual, hasty, repetitive manner, but only with relaxed, creative and prolonged erotic practice. Mindful Masturbation can take you into high quality states of extended erotic trance comparable with the whole body/brain ecstasies of psychedelic drugs administered in carefully guided conditions.

However, this erotic practice produces intense, ongoing states of body/brain ecstasy without the often overwhelming and uncontrollable hallucinatory aspects of psychedelics. At the same time, this natural process can definitely produce mystical altered states of profound visionary and revelatory experience, of a life-enhancing, life-affirming, and life-changing quality.

Mindful Masturbation can actually wire new neural pathways through processes now understood as "neuroplasticity," and "epigenetics." This not only adds complexity to your brain and nervous system, it also influences what chromosomes are activated and which are inhibited throughout your trillions of cells. Your reality is changed.

The process is capable of harmoniously orchestrating the incredibly complex symphony of your embodied existence, to naturally optimize your internal body functions of circulation, respiration, digestion, elimination, heart rate, blood pressure, neurochemistry and hormonal balances.

This is not a process you control consciously, rather you create the circumstances for its possibility, and allow it to happen naturally according to innate potentials of your body/mind system—when you get out of your own way.

There is no limit to where this can take you with a willingness to explore.

Though your conscious mind may have forgotten it, this is the secret that you already know deep inside, when you listen to what your body tells you is possible.

It is the cellular wisdom of your ancestors that goes back several billion years to the dawn of DNA; it is the atomic, stardust wisdom of your universal ancestry that emerged some 13.7 billion years ago with the Universe itself in the event we call the Big Bang.

Male Erotic Alchemy provides you with access to this limitless potential you already have, which only awaits awakening and activation from within you, in order to transform you and your life.

The Phallic Serpent

Perhaps the most common and essential phallic symbol among archetypes is the Serpent. An archetype is a basic, powerful, universal symbol not bound by the specific limitations of any particular culture; it has a literal and experiential quality. It represents something that any human individual might experience, regardless of background or location.

Most of the stories of phallic mythology in this book include Serpent imagery. In every case you may consider these Phallic Serpents to represent your penis or some aspect of its power and significance.

The overall resemblance of your penis to an actual snake is obvious: a generally tubular creature with a distinct head and a tailend. It's a flexibly muscular and versatile form. Despite having been vilified or reviled by some, this Phallic Serpent is a creature of priceless value and is worthy of worship.

The correspondences go far beyond the purely physical parallels, compelling enough in themselves to give any observer pause. However the qualities I call "deeper and higher," of your penis and the Phallic Serpent are that they resonate with core aspects of how the Universe is organized.

Both literally in your experience and as an archetypal image, the Serpent has an ancient biological relationship with your primate ancestors. Clearly humans have some degree of hard-wired fear of stepping on a snake. Even a person who has friendly relations with the limbless slithering varieties of our herpetological kin, may react instinctively with a start when the twisted root of a tree, or a fallen bit of rope first catches peripheral vision. We tend to jump or feel startled. This is a deep instinct.

A rush of adrenaline and a jolt of cortisol surges from your brain through your body. Immediately when you realize that you have *not* almost stepped on a snake—you probably laugh at yourself. Yet your heart will still beat swiftly with the afterglow of the fight/flight reflex that has been triggered!

Penile arousal, the Living Phallus that stands up from between your legs, is allied with the relaxation response, the other portion of your autonomic nervous system that functions apart from the alarmed, stressful, reaction-oriented portion. These aspects, the relaxation response and the fight/flight response are actual physical parts of your nervous system, wired-in with two quite different patterns into the overall structure of your spinal column.

Your spine forms the trunk of the "Tree of Life" that is your central nervous system comprising brain and spinal column. Your brain can be compared with the canopy of the tree, having branches and leafy crown. The Serpent Power of Yoga ascends the spinal column from root to crown in your torso. The Serpent of the Garden Story is associated with the major trees of Paradise, and is actually the Phallic Serpent.

Once you begin to look for the Phallic Serpent, it reveals itself in many forms. Every vertical axis, such as the letter "I," can be seen as the phallus or trunk of the tree.

The symbol for Phallic Brotherhood is comprised of an oval, egg-shaped version of the ancient Greek image of Ouroboros, or the "Serpent that bites its own tail." This Ouroboros encloses within its inner region the "Hieroglyphic Monad" invented and described by Dr. John Dee, a scholar, Magus and Alchemist of Elizabethan times. This universal sign includes all basic numbers, elements, planetary and zodiacal signs condensed into a single glyph. Dee considered it a universal image of the cosmic order.

You are created in the image of the Universe.

Dee's Monad offers an embryonic image of universal symbology.

The Monad graphically depicts the nature of phallic power on all levels including your erect penis itself, your entire body, and the whole Universe—all of which have corresponding forms of organization and functional integrity.

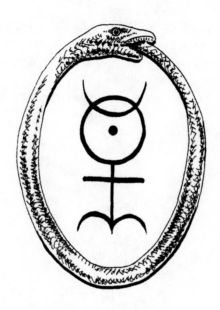

Phallic Brotherhood Logo

This fascinating glyph returns later in this book just as the Ouroboros forever returns to swallow its own tail without beginning or end as an image of masturbatory self-love, self-reference, and constant creation.

Ouroboros enclosing the glyph perfectly represents the literal reality of you as a mindful masturbator, in continual self-reference, manipulating and stimulating your erection with full attention and ever-expanding awareness of the transformational potency of pure penile pleasure. This Serpent is also the microcosmic orbit of erotic energy that moves through your body while in arousal, down your front as you breath and up your back to your head in a constant, ongoing cycle.

As you masturbate mindfully, you not only experience higher quality and more prolonged erotic sensations than ever before; it resembles the musical feedback produced by a talented electric guitarist. The ecstasy generates brain chemicals and hormones that can re-imprint you with lasting therapeutic benefits. With practice and dedication you can recreate yourself and become a happier, healthier and more balanced man.

Within your own body, legally, naturally and safely, you are capable of generating neurochemistry and hormonal balances that can produce permanent beneficial changes to how your feel and function from now on.

Your penis is a remarkably complex, highly evolved organ of communication and communion with your inner self, capable of taking you on the ultimate trip—the journey of the rest of your lifetime lived as a well-adjusted, sane and mature human male.

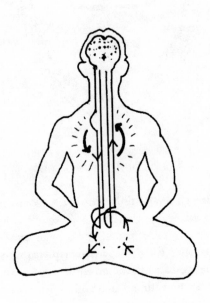

Two-Way Flow of Signals between Genitals and Brain

What Yogis call the Serpent Power, is not merely a metaphysical idea. In reality this is the two-way flow of signals that traverse your spinal column between your genitals and your brain, an ongoing traffic of bliss to illuminate your torso, and light up your entire body. Your heart is located as the central "traffic circle" of this flow of signals between root and crown.

The blissful fluidity of feeling totally alive opens your heart to loving yourself better with each breath, and with every beat of your heart. By this same process you can also better love others.

The True Nature of Your Phallic Power

During the last few thousand years limiting beliefs about the penis have proliferated along with the male dominant culture. Why is this so? This is because male leaders dominate other men in order to dominate everyone else. This has been effectively accomplished with unnatural controls on the sexuality of males, by imposing certain taboos and superstitions.

Male erotic energy has been hidden and limited in order to control men. The true nature of your phallic power has been obscured. It has become "occulted," which means hidden. Yet now, the time for such secrecy and hiding is over!

Humanity has learned to associate male sexuality with patriarchal societies in which armed warriors intimidate and enforce the agendas of male rulers. Men control and own women, and perpetuate their lineage by reproducing themselves through their sons and designated heirs. Men have become obsessively goal-oriented and have forgotten the benefits of prolonged ecstasy. Businessmen are often too busy for real pleasure!

In practice countless men experience the qualities of conditioned "masculinity," as if they were natural and inevitable: a heart shielded from strong emotions, a mind in control of the body and its urges. Plus a need to compete with other males for control of possessions, resources and power. A suspicion of sensitivity and feelings, as if they are signs of weakness, when in reality quite the opposite is true!

As such, phallic power has attained a false reputation as oppressive, controlling, dominant and even destructive. Indeed, its falsification has had *actual* dire consequences. None of these negative qualities are natural and inevitable in relation to the living phallus.

In reality, genuine and natural phallic power has nothing to do with power over anyone or anything else, rather it is the creative male energy. It is power from within you. Such phallic power is lively, energetic, enthusiastic, and playful, tender and tough. It is sensitive in its strength, as the erect penis is both strong and sensitive. This inherent biological power of potency and enthusiasm inspires you to drop any pretense, and to celebrate your actual nature as a human male animal. In essence you are naturally loving, and nurturing, as well as playful and strong.

Make no mistake—there is nothing wimpy or passive about actual peace. Peace is a state of dynamic integrity and harmony, based on love, rather than the fearful and insecure paradigm that motivates conflict and warfare.

Peace is genuine strength.

Inner peace is real freedom, of a kind that no other person can give you or take away from you. Peaceful surroundings emanate from the peace you cultivate within you.

Peace comes from confidence, inner balance, and a sense of total aliveness.

To cultivate the phallic energy through erotic ecstasy, to re-connect the brain/mind with the genitals, is the most effective way to re-open the shielded male heart, to achieve inner peace, and to connect with others in a balanced manner.

In this sense we are all walking wounded. Our hearts become shielded by personal history and conditioning. The male heart almost inevitably disconnects from both genitals and brain. Human males in today's world are often shattered, fragmented creatures. Men in our global civilization tend to suffer touch deprivation, and an inability to love the self.

Erotic ecstasy of sustained high quality can heal these wounds.

The true phallic power, of creativity, love and integrity, is many times more powerful than the fear-based male-dominant lies of conditioned "masculinity."

You need not take this on faith; your own experience will confirm the true nature of your phallic power.

True phallic power is creative, sustaining, and regenerative.
Phallic power is the way to recover your true self.
You are your penis; your penis is you.

Your Natural and Biological Inheritance

You are the heir to a priceless fortune that continues to expand. With each beat of your heart, your inherited wealth expands faster than it expanded during your previous heartbeat. Rather than losing anything, with each moment the richness of your existence increases.

Your body manifests a design that reflects the design principles of the Universe itself. You are a product of Nature. You are an animal, which is not an insult; rather it's an honor and a great gift! Your animal nature is in fact a priceless asset.

Matter is reality; your body exists as a natural part of the material Universe, whose deeper nature is the ceaseless, timeless dance of energy.

The 100 billion neurons of your brain, along with the virtually numberless connections among those neurons, comprise a truly remarkable brain and nervous system. Each and every ultra-sensitive pleasure-receptor nerve of your remarkably evolved, and sophisticated human penis is directly connected with your brain and your entire nervous system.

Your penis has been evolving for many millions of years, plus its rate of evolution has accelerated during the several million years of evolution of our own species. As the planet's evolution now goes exponential, so must the evolution of your penis, which is the key to your conscious evolution overall. Otherwise you could get left behind…

This rate of adaptive evolution continues to accelerate.

Now on a planet and at a time when over-population pressures generate deep-seated problems for all species, the nature of human male sexuality has evolved beyond recognition. Males of our species always hunger for physical, recreational pleasure, and there is nothing wrong with this. In fact, we're designed and hard-wired this way. Pure penile pleasure may be deliberately separated from the reproductive process.

We're at a turning point when the urge to reproduce must no longer be automatically sanctioned, rather it needs to be questioned, possibly redirected toward recreational eroticism, and healthy alternatives offered with encouragement.

Reproduction must be rendered a conscious, careful process for the sake of quality of life on Earth. Same-sex recreational eroticism between human males should be encouraged for the benefit of all people, all creatures and the living environments of the planet. Males have a strong desire for physical pleasure, which is healthy.

This proposition to encourage male same-sex play is a practical necessity, in order to stop merely treating the symptoms of our deep-rooted problems, and to directly treat the causes. Human males have been handed a huge set of false assumptions concerning the nature of masculinity and manhood. Conditioned agreements concerning the nature of things passed on by both caretakers and context, assume the virtue and necessity of heterosexual relationships and that reproductive agenda called "the nuclear family."

Current evidence indicates that the two-parent family unit and monogamous, exclusively heterosexual relationships are often *not* the most effective patterns for human beings to practice. Children benefit from an extended family of honorary "aunts" and "uncles" as caretakers and mentors along with their biological parents. In most tribal and hunter-gatherer cultures—aside from missionary influences—exclusive monogamy is not expected, and sexuality is far more fluid. Any adult may have significant erotic relationships with at least several lovers, quite often of both sexes.

Monogamy, marriage and monotheism tend to go hand-in-hand. These concepts were created partly to foster the increase of human populations for the purpose of plentiful agricultural workers, and the expendable military personnel called guards and soldiers. Patriarchal kings clamped down upon the importance of the mother goddesses in order to exert control over women and children as property. Plus they required the unquestioning loyalty of warriors willing to fight and die to protect the culture and its patriarchal values.

Older men sacrificed young men to enact their agendas, and conditioned the masses of people to believe this is not only inevitable, but also noble and natural.

Obedience to authority, marital subservience, and slavery, are among the less desirable inventions of the patriarchal paradigm—still patriarchy has not been all bad. During the several thousand years of patriarchy and monotheism, much good has also been accomplished. Many aspects of collective culture, centralized cooperation, and communication benefit everyone.

However, now the legacy of patriarchy must be seriously questioned.

Through the astounding agency of DNA you have inherited the physiological design of a male human body. Until recently the dominant belief in genetic determinism suggested that we humans are basically biological robots, controlled by the DNA in the nuclei of our cells. The new understanding of epigenetics has overturned this belief. Your environment as well as your experience and behavior, constantly influences which chromosomes in your cells are expressed, and which are inhibited.

Everything you experience, both external and internal is forever switching on and off various chromosomes among the trillions of cells of your body. Every bit as astonishing is the fact that your human body IS a collective organism, a collaboration of life forms that are actually too numerous, too constantly-evolving to imagine.

In fact, each nucleated cell of your body is like a super-computer mini-universe far more complex and integrated than anything humans can create via technology. The microbial forms that co-habit with your human cells, and co-create the collective entity you consider to be "you," actually out-number those inherent body cells ten-to-one! In other words, multiply the roughly 100 trillion cells of your body ten times to estimate the microbial "population" of your collective organism!

When you sustain erotic ecstasy at high levels indefinitely with artful masturbatory or erotic skill, all of those biological entities, each cell, every molecule, all the atoms of stardust and the dance of energies composing them, light up with the mysterious and powerful glow of awareness. This bliss illuminates your ten-to-one microbial cohorts as well! The synergy generated is truly beyond imagining.

The complexity and creative potential of the body vehicle you inherit from your ancestors is like a starship that is also a time machine. Will you use it to go to the corner convenience store for a few standard pre-packaged, processed food necessities? That is what happens if you settle for an ordinary, predictable, repetitive sex life!

And yet the reality is that you live in the Garden of Paradise; you are the New Adam of the New Earth.

Your body IS the holy temple in which you can honor the Source of Life and the Universe and Powers without any other intermediary. Far more than a mere temporary dwelling place, this sacred body can serve as a portal to literally return you to your lost state of Original Innocence, the actual Eden, to embrace your own divinity.

Living becomes Heaven on Earth.

The cumulative energy of the male ancestry within you stands behind your phallus and its remarkable qualities as an organ of inner awareness, outer communication, and phallic communion with fellow humans.

Your phallic power emerges from the vitality and beauty of literally thousands of male ancestors, millions of years of human evolution, more than 3.5 billion years of biological evolution, plus about 13.7 billion years of evolving stardust.

Be the King of Your Life

Despite how acquired assumptions may cloud the issue, nothing can be more spiritual than the full embrace of your sacred embodiment. Your body is a gift from the Source of All Things, equivalent to the mystery of existence itself.

All religions and cultures contain much wisdom and beliefs that can enhance the lives of believers. Along the way all traditions have also acquired some ambivalence and often, definite negativity concerning human sexuality.

Experience teaches that you have your own direct connection with Source. Plus change for the better only comes about through inner transformation, when you make a choice to surrender to the greater good. This shift happens when you are willing to shed all those "outer layers" of the things that are not your authentic self, in favor of total authenticity.

Your basic physical heritage as an embodied human male arrives genetically. Yet the set of concepts that are often considered natural "masculinity," upon close examination turns out to be arbitrary and about 99% invalid.

Those qualities designated "feminine" prove every bit as arbitrary and false. Without exception, all such qualities—so-called masculine and so-called feminine—form at least some part of every human individual's qualities. More accurate terms are simply male and female, which have a literal biological basis.

Every person is incredibly complex, mysterious, inexplicable and contradictory.

At the same time, on a certain level, a human male is incredibly simple.

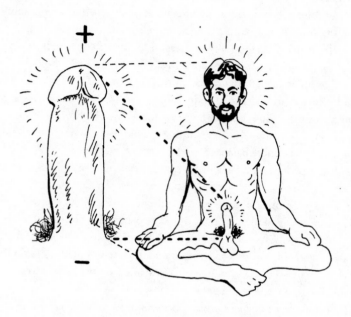

The Microcosm and the Macrocosm

Your penis is a smaller version of the whole of you, and you as a whole are a larger version of your penis. Your penis is a microcosm of you, and you are the macrocosm of your penis. Through Penis Reflexology—detailed later in this book—you discover that this is more than theoretical. The correspondences and direct connections can be experienced.

You are your penis; your penis is you.

Any objections that arise within you to such an honest and liberating statement of truth are issues worth examining.

At present, an important consideration is the most effective way to let go of those invalid beliefs and assumptions made *for* you by others. The most effective means is to accept 100% responsibility for everything that shows up in your reality: *no exceptions!*

This does not mean you should feel any guilt or blame—on the contrary. At the same time, literally everything in your awareness shows up because in some way you participate in its creation. You are a co-creator of all that you experience.

You discover to your astonishment, that with 100% responsibility is total freedom! When you no longer blame anyone or anything outside of yourself for anything, ironically that responsibility sets you free. It allows you to let go of any form of victimhood. This is the ultimate self-empowerment.

Now apply this 100% responsibility to your attitude toward your penis, and to the quality and the quantity of erotic ecstasy you cultivate via pure penile pleasure. When you begin to experience this kind of freedom from the need to blame or control anyone or anything else, you become incredibly powerful and far more balanced and happy than ever before.

You experience the reality that erotic ecstasy is limitless. Ecstasy is the process of creative energy itself at a universal level. Though you may seem to come and go from it, limitless ecstasy is always present. With this realization, you neither cling to pleasure nor push away pain and suffering.

This is the nature of your phallic liberation: you can allow the full intensity and range of embodied experience to flow through you like a river. This flow nourishes and cleanses you constantly: it's the great adventure of feeling totally alive in your body!

As the ecstatic energy circulates between your root and crown, the two-way traffic not only restores the open and feeling capacities of your heart—it also eventually opens what yogis call the "thousand-petalled lotus" at the top of your head, which connects you with transpersonal or universal realities.

You enjoy ever-expanding awareness that connects you with All Things. Separation is seen for the lie and illusion that it has always been!

As the circuit of ecstatic energy that circulates through your torso renders you a happier, more balanced human male, you become the King of your own Life.

As such, to be a King simply means that you govern your own existence from the natural nobility of your genetic origins as a human male, in full possession of your phallic power that connects you with every aspect of your inherent realm.

How to Be an Incarnate Phallic God

Sustained, high quality pure penile pleasure gradually burns away your sense of ordinary mortal individuality and leaves you feeling purified, cleansed and refined to your essential nature as a phallic god. The ordinary limitations of space and time dissolve. You feel connected with everything: One with All Things.

Your body, your genitals, your erection, your entire being expresses the Divine.

The importance of your individual personality and egoic identity diminishes, and the sense of separation, which is the cause of all suffering, also gradually dissolves. Boundaries soften. You can identify all phenomena as arising and passing forms that emerge from Source and dissolve back into Source without urgency.

From deep within you this awareness emerges: ***Nothing is actually separate from anything else.***

Your activated, charged phallus provides you with the direct experience of creative energy as it flows—what we call the Universe is really only that experience of flowing and circulating energy. Your aroused phallus itself acts as an organ of non-dual awareness—the energetic *seeing* of Oneness.

To *see* in this manner is not merely visual sight, but full awareness: to sense and to know with your entire body and being.

Oneness simply IS; you are already there. You are *always* there. You cannot enter or leave Oneness, or achieve Oneness. It's all that exists. It simply IS.

On the deeper levels of your cells, your DNA, and your stardust, you know this. You have always known this deep inside. It is who and what you truly are.

This awareness is not a process of discovery, so much as remembering something your conscious mind easily forgets.

By practicing Mindful Masturbation you awaken from within your cells the awareness that you are a phallic god. This is what your male human body is designed for, not only to benefit you, but also all of humanity and the planet. The ancestral phallic power within you, and the connection with your phallic brothers in the world around you, is your true essential identity.

As a phallic god you may also serve to inspire your fellow men to cultivate their erotic potential. Yet it begins with you. It begins with the full, conscious embrace of your phallic power, its sacred origins and Divine nature.

Re-discover this power that is already inside of you.

You *are* the divinity you have been seeking.

Look between your legs and *see*.

CHAPTER TWO:

PHALLIC CREATION MYTHS DEPICT YOUR BODY

Mythology provides stories and images that illustrate aspects of the world of your experience and possible explanations of what important aspects of that world may mean. Myths offer insight into the nature of the self and the environment, plus the capital-S Self of the Divine, plus how all these may be related.

Some myths explain the origins of the world and its features and qualities. Others illustrate key relationships, such as parents and children or humans and Nature.

Mythic archetypes are images, relationships or stories that convey essential patterns of meaning, so universal that they are not bound to any one culture. Archetypes hold immense potency because they are also shared by all of humanity through our unconscious minds, which seem to tap into a collective reservoir of imagery and significance.

At any rate, though we may feel our conscious mind controls things, in fact the much deeper, vaster unconscious mind is where all that we experience actually comes from.

The conscious mind is that portion of your awareness that seems to deliberately think and perceive what is going on. However the conscious mind in itself provides an extremely limited version of reality.

Most of the contents of the conscious mind simply bubble up into awareness like effervescence from the far vaster, totally mysterious and unknown unconscious mind. This emergence occurs without your deliberate choice. You do not create it consciously.

In a sense your conscious awareness simply happens.

Plus, operating from the conscious mind is like peering through a tiny fish-eye lens and mistaking that distorted view for reality. This limited version of what is going on is mediated by the brain processing about *forty bits of information per second.*

The immense, oceanic, chaotic and magickal realm of the unconscious mind, which includes all the rest of the brain processes, along with the entire central nervous system, and peripheral nerve networks throughout the body, processes about *forty million bits per second!*

Thus that unconscious mind—which cannot actually be controlled or tamed in any way—plays a far greater role than the conscious mind does in creating your reality. Its functioning processes outnumber the conscious mind by *about a million-to-one!*

You cannot presume to control or tame this unconscious mind. Even less can you master or direct the collective realm that all of humanity seems to share as ocean life shares its oceanic home from the sunny surface to the deepest lightless depths... however, this is not bad news. Rather, it simply means that effective function is less along the lines of control and more along the lines of navigation and cooperation.

The unconscious mind is like a deeper and higher dimension of data that describes all possible archetypal elements, beings, and stories, in an undifferentiated churning, circulating, stream of currents, eddies and whirlpools.

Jules Verne's famous fictional character, Captain Nemo, an East Indian nobleman of truly Renaissance talents, created the archetypal submarine, the *Nautilus*, that appears in the early sci-fi novels *Twenty Thousand Leagues Under the Sea* and *The Mysterious Island*. Like the *Nautilus* your activated and energized phallus allows you to travel through and navigate the unconscious realm, which otherwise may prove bewildering in scope, and sometimes even seems dangerous.

However, when you grasp this reality that the thoughts you think merely percolate into your conscious awareness like boiling water that spurts up and brews coffee in an old-fashioned stovetop percolator, you realize that your conscious mind is a most mysterious island that rises from a far deeper sea than you may have thought.

All mythologies, the various beings such as spirits, ghosts, monsters, demi-gods, deities, families and pantheons of gods, even the monotheistic Creator God, all actually represent processes within your own body on levels of the biological organs, the cells, constituent molecules, and the atoms of stardust that compose them.

In terms of mythic significance, the beings and worlds depicted by various mythologies can be interpreted as "maps" or "story diagrams" of your body and of the universal human design your body reflects.

The Prehistoric Origins of Phallic Veneration

From long before the dawn of history, which is usually considered the first written records—perhaps created by the ancient Sumerians, circa. 3400 BCE—human beings have venerated their own bodies and generative organs as images of divinity, as well as the source of abundance in Nature.

Circular and spiral patterns, along with triangular designs are often interpreted as goddess imagery, for their general resemblance to breasts and vulvas. The phallus associated with a phallic god is often far less ambiguous, even in the simplest representations. The association with a deity is usually far less certain.

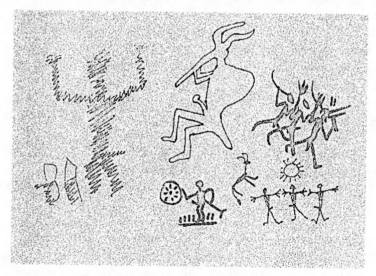

Prehistoric Phallic Art

Artwork and artifacts that depict the phallus and men with erections go back many millennia, in the form of pictographic drawings inscribed onto rock surfaces, carvings of stone, bone, and wood, and paintings on the walls of caves. Goddess-oriented scholars sometimes claim that the female form, including breasts and vulvas are the earliest sacred images, and there is no reason to argue this point. Most such interpretations cannot really be proven one way or another.

Still, the earliest beliefs that we can reconstruct usually involve a Great Mother Goddess and her consort, a Horned God, who are the divine parents of All Things.

Clearly, prehistoric humans, like their modern descendents, were fascinated with human bodies and genitalia.

Human sexuality was also identified with fertility in Nature—the reproduction of animals and the growth cycles of vegetation. The connection is valid and natural to make, for it has literal reality. Our own reproductive and regenerative processes resemble and correspond with those of creatures and plants.

We are directly related to all life forms on Earth through genetic descent from common ancestry.

Prehistoric art not only shows the erect penis itself as a sacred image of male creative and regenerative power, but groups of men sporting erections. Stick figures in groups, every one of them ithyphallic—a word that means "with a straight or erect phallus"—suggest that these groups of men shared what we call the Male Mysteries. In some cases the men appear to engage in group masturbation.

Into historic times, similar images have continued to appear, though with the rise of the patriarchal, male dominant societies that use homophobia as a control mechanism, such imagery grows scarcer.

Egyptian graffiti or informal wall art includes groups of men, all of them ithyphallic, celebrating the joys of masturbating together.

Where intolerance rules, such groups of men masturbating together must often conduct such Male Mysteries in a secretive manner. Yet an honest take on human nature makes it clear that similar gatherings have doubtless occurred quite often, at least in private, for many millennia.

In fact, such rituals of a group masturbatory nature have probably occurred fairly often ever since the earliest proto-human males assumed an upright bipedal stance and took notice of the possibilities several million years ago. Standing on two legs with clearly visible genitals at the middle, in front and within convenient reach of clever hands obviously adds up!

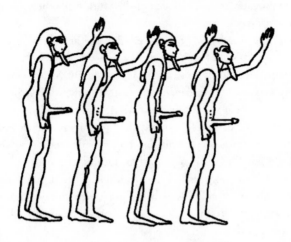

Egyptian Erotic Graffiti

We know little of the specific practices such Male Mystery groups engaged in. Except we do know that humans have also gathered around fires since around 1.5 million years ago, generally facing one another, ever since humans began to build such fires for warmth and cooking purposes. It's natural for human groups to form circles around a central fire in which every individual has a direct view of all the other individuals.

What later cultures often came to view as symbolic abstractions, removed a step or many steps from actuality, earlier cultures viewed and experienced as direct, actual practices.

Tune in to those male ancestors within you. These men will tell you they always loved to masturbate, and in many cases they loved to masturbate with fellow men. They enjoyed mutual masturbation with fellow human males, and probably frottage as well. Meanwhile the women were occupied with the Female Mysteries such as their synchronized menstrual cycles, childbirth, and their maiden, mother and crone initiation rituals.

Such prehistoric cultures most often employed both gathering and hunting strategies to provide their food and useful materials. We base these interpretations on surviving hunter-gatherers, as well as archaeological evidence. In many cases the hunters were groups of men who periodically left the home base on hunting expeditions, while the women and children remained at the home base. Everyone did some gathering, however women and children probably often did much of this work while the men went off on hunting expeditions together.

Those groups of hunters probably enacted the first formalized phallic rites of the Male Mysteries. While temporarily isolated from their kin, the all-male groups most likely practiced collective masturbatory rituals both for solidarity and in order to contact the animal spirits of their prey. Their sexuality remained fluid and flexible. The warriors gained individual balance and the group gained collective harmony through this erotic male bonding.

In such tribal societies, to this day no separation exists between the material world and the spiritual realm. Everything is done in the sacred manner, as this is the only way to do everything. Though modern people often romanticize tribal cultures as being model environmental stewards, this is not always the case. In reality many tribal people usually kill and eat anything they can catch.

At the same time the close connection with Nature and Spirit are indeed aspects of tribal cultures that we as modern techno-humans have lost and that are important connections for us to reclaim. The new identity as an "Ecosexual" allows people of any sexual orientation to identify their erotic energy with treating the Earth and Nature itself as a beloved lover.

Now, as global humans we can also define the male spiritual warrior as a man on a spiritual path who employs love as his only weapon.

Contemporary men of our often fragmented, isolated, and yet electronically interwoven civilization can benefit by reclaiming the Male Mysteries to recover balance and group harmony through the rites of Phallic Brotherhood.

This is not theoretical: let's *do* it! At the end of this book you'll find resources and connections to actually participate in this new erotic revolution. Today, the erotic Male Mystery School has sprung back to life, so check it out and consider participating!

Origins—the Seed Source Stories

Imagine: Your body is a Universe; your head is filled with stars, galaxies and nebulas of symbolic constellations; your heart beats incessantly like the Sun shining its steady radiance from the center of the local solar system;

your navel is a maternal connection at the middle that links you directly with the Earth; your penis is like the Moon, with an endless cycle of lunar waxing and waning.

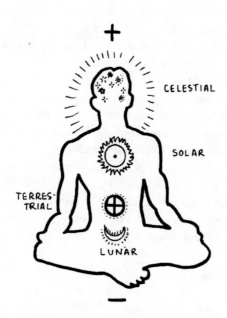

Your Body viewed as a Universe

Such phallic/lunar power is cyclical, regenerative and transformational.

Both Moon and phallus go through repeating cycles. Both relate to the tidal cycles of surging liquid and emotional intensity that wax and wane repeatedly and incessantly. Plus both the lunar orb and your penis bear important relations to other cycles of growth, flourishing and renewal throughout the natural world.

Like the Serpent—also a phallic symbol for obvious reasons—the lunar cycle is considered one of emergence into form, development, dissolving back, and then being regenerated to continue the cycle. The Serpent periodically sheds its skin as it grows.

As the true nature of the phallic power has already been identified with creative power, confidence, strength, sensitivity, bliss and life-enhancement, many ancient creation myths, regardless of the culture, have strong elements of phallic imagery.

Most of the early phallic gods were either a Sky Father, or a Rain God, such as Indra, Menu, Uranus, Zeus, Odin, Thor, Kokopelli, Itzamna, and Tlaloc. These deities and their brethren brought life-giving rainfall down from Above, and inspired the upward growth of vegetation from Below. Sometimes the rain with its attendant fertile growth was considered the silvery semen of such celestial deities that poured down to bestow life force and abundance upon the world.

The scientific theory of "panspermia" suggests that life on Earth may have extraterrestrial origins—not that the "seeding with Life" was necessarily deliberate. Still there is a variation of the concept that is called "directed panspermia," which indicates deliberate seeding by some agent or agency. This could even take the form of the innate properties of matter at the quantum level that give rise to life, or beings of advanced intelligence capable of deliberately broadcasting the Starseed through the cosmos.

The potentials for planetary life may exist within the nature of stardust itself, those complex atoms necessary for the existence of our biosphere.

Stardust as such did not emerge directly from the Big Bang, which expanded and cooled to produce mostly hydrogen and helium atoms. Rather stardust only appeared with the first generation of stars that were born, lived and died in cataclysmic explosions. In the hearts of those ancient stars such complex atoms as carbon and iron—necessary for biological Life as we know it—were created. Then the supernova explosions that destroyed those ancestral stars broadcast the stardust for the formation of later generations of stars and planetary systems.

Our own Sun is a third generation star, its stardust cycled through two prior generations. As a precursor for life, such stardust has sometimes been called the Starseed.

Possibly, planetary life arises whenever the Starseed encounters certain conditions for its innate potentials to unfold. On Earth the emergence of amino acids led to nucleic acids, cells, and multi-celled collective organisms such as me and you.

Because the Starseed apparently provides the origin and genetic blueprints for the entire biosphere of a living planet, it has a phallic quality, just as the phallus is the creative source and provides the patterns for living forms.

The Story of Uranus and Gaia

The same basic idea as the scientific theory of panspermia is also found in ancient myths of a "Sky Father and Virginal Planetary Goddess" such as the ancient Greek story of Uranus and Gaia…

The virginal, childless goddess Gaia languishes in space, beautiful, fully formed and yet devoid of life, and lonely. Her longing for both companionship and children reaches into the starry cosmos and attracts to her the Star Prince, or Lord of the Sky, named Uranus. He descends to her untouched surface, accepts her invitation and impregnates Gaia with all the subsequent generations that will be born from her body.

Almost immediately, she begins to give birth, and his promiscuous gaze wanders to other conquests. As Sky Fathers always do, Uranus soon begins to play the field, and he seeks other conquests. Gaia's first children are her Beloved Monsters, the oldest primordial forces of Nature seen as giants, dragons and chimeras.

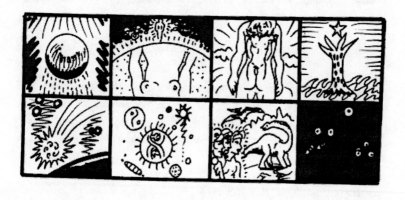

Gaia's Beloved Monsters are born and banished

The following generation is the group of elder gods we call Titans. They are not so monstrous and look more like their father in basic appearance, thus Uranus favors them.

However Gaia loves all of her children, whether monstrous or fair. She will only favor any of them in order to restore balance if some are oppressed by others. So when Uranus banishes the Monsters to the dark underworld of Tartarus simply because he finds them hideous, Gaia complains to him. He promises that he will soon release her Beloved Monsters back into the surface world... only he never does.

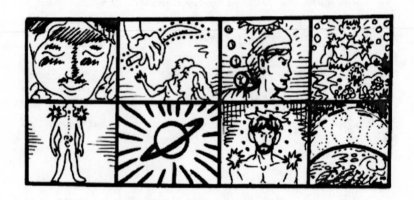

Gaia helps Kronus overthrow Uranus

Thus Gaia helps her son Kronus, the eldest Titan, by giving him a stone sickle so that he can overthrow his father. Kronus has promised his mother Gaia that he will release her Beloved Monsters, whose unhappy struggles in Tartarus produce terrible earthquakes and violent volcanic eruptions on the surface. So Kronus tracks down his father, uses the sickle to emasculate him, and tosses his severed testicles into the ocean.

The injured Uranus flees back to the Sky, his original realm, while the semen that gushes from his testicles into the ocean becomes the white frothy foam on the waves, where it engenders Aphrodite. The Goddess of Love appears naked and alluring, standing upright upon the foam, as she drifts to the shoreline.

Though Gaia hopes that Kronus will be true to his word, he in turn fails to release her Beloved Monsters, so again in turn she covertly helps his eldest son, Zeus, to overthrow Kronus. Thus begins the rule of the Olympian gods—and it seems that Gaia's troubles with her children have proven perennial...

Here's the universal archetype: The male seed-energy comes down vertically from Above, conceives and engenders generations of living things in the female realm of matter Below, then returns vertically to the Above. This becomes a cycle and a circulation of energy.

Because your phallus stands "upright" with the erection of your penis, your phallic energy aligns with the vertical axis on the planetary surface.

In parallel, when you stand upright as a man, your spine and entire body aligns with this axis that connects Below and Above. Your body is a biological form of this axis, and your erect penis expresses the same vertical connection. This verticality does not defy gravity, rather it balances *upon* gravity, precisely as the growth of vegetation does, rising from roots to the apex of growth. *This does not challenge or dominate the female nature of matter, rather it harmonizes and cooperates with its qualities.*

To return to the imagery of science for a moment, what we call the Big Bang is also represented in many creation myths as a kind of primordial ejaculation.

Your erections and orgasmic sensations literally replay that cosmic origin and likewise involve you and your body with a weave of creative mythic scenarios.

The phallic significance for you: While you masturbate, pay close attention to the deepest and highest awareness within you. The oldest stories of Creation are all encoded within your stardust, from which the molecules of your DNA are composed, and which evolves through your ancestry into the fabulous cellular architecture of your male body and genitals.

Your body is a Universe of such complexity that you cannot begin to comprehend it; rather more useful is simply to honor and surrender to its powerful mystery. Those Beloved Monsters of Gaia, her first children are really the oldest primordial forces of Nature. They are immense ancient powers and instincts within you that exist in your unconscious mind, and it's a good idea to honor and embrace them.

During your enjoyment of phallic arousal, notice the difference between lying down while you masturbate, and standing up to masturbate.

Don't think about it too much—simply notice your sensations and enjoy.

The Phallic Forest and the Horned God

A tall, awe-inspiring figure moves through dappled light and shade of the forest floor, where he pauses, and then he moves onward again. The lean form ripples with muscle and he sports a huge erection that wobbles stiffly as he moves. His wide clear eyes on the bearded face drink in everything around him.

This woodland god Pançika roams the Phallic Forest naked and aroused. His mere presence and the potency of his divine phallus inspires the growth of the vegetation on every side. Pançika wears nothing but a headdress with horns, which also connects him with the virility of male animals, such as the bull and the stag.

In this primeval forest, all of the trees and green things that grow upward toward the Sun reflect the power of this phallic god, and in this way they all resemble erect penises. His divine phallus inspires not only the growth and form of the mighty trees, but every green and growing thing as well as phallus-shaped mushrooms.

Humans who enter this woodland to ask for Pançika's blessings of fertility and bliss are welcome so long as they respect his sacred realm and his Male Mysteries.

In the Phallic Forest you find no stories of conflict or struggle, no drama beyond the natural cycles of growth and regeneration, feeding and predation, recycling and cooperation among various species.

Pançika has the apparent form of a strong, virile, erect human male; however in reality he is a being of Nature itself, and serves the Great Mother of All Life.

This early imagery stems from the ancient Indus Valley culture that flourished along the rivers of what are now southern Pakistan and northern India.

The original deity called Pançika, Protector of Animals, was the consort of a many-breasted Mother Nature Goddess named Hariti. Pançika is an early form of the primordial Lord of Yogis, the Mountain God, depicted on seals from the Indus Valley (circa. 2800 BCE). The Mountain God is shown as a male figure that sits naked and cross-legged; he wears a headdress with horns, and sports an erect phallus. He has three faces that represent his three aspects: creative, sustaining, and regenerative.

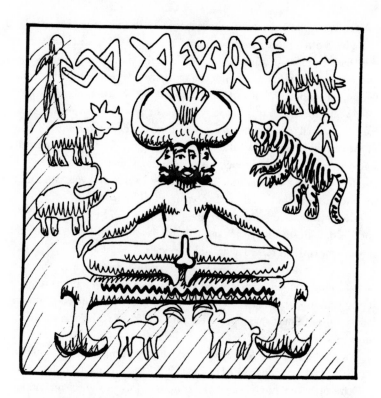

The Mountain God: Protector of Animals and Lord of Yogis

The earliest images of the Mountain God derive from incised cylinder seals that were rolled across moist clay to produce an image. Though many details of the image, including his identification as the Mountain God are somewhat debatable, this book is not a work of scholarly argument. Rather, when ancient phallic gods are considered it is important to accept feedback from your own cellular wisdom and to allow information from the deepest and highest levels within you and without you to fill in gaps. This helps you to assess speculative unknowns.

For example, the earliest depictions of the Horned Mountain God from the Indus Valley culture show him as a seated male figure with three faces or three heads, which connects him with the important Triple God archetype about which a great deal more is offered in the following chapters.

This image has not changed in essence over the millennia. Later, as Lord Shiva he is often shown seated similarly cross-legged. He wears only a tiger skin, has a cobra draped around his neck, and the "horns" appear as the lunar crescent perched on his head. You can recognize in these features the animal nature, the Serpent Power and the lunar qualities of a classical phallic god.

While we have no detailed narrative or plot that involves the early Pançika, a phallic principle emerges of him wandering the Phallic Forest Primeval. His presence and the power of his erection emanate the creative seed-energy at work all through his surroundings, and provide both energy and form for the living growth. At the deepest level within you, this forest is the ancient home to the arboreal ancestors of all humans.

In fact, the Greek woodland deity the Great God Pan, Lord of Forest and Field, with strikingly similar attributes, is a form of Pançika, who thus traveled far without really changing his essence.

Pançika embodies the vibrant life force that drives vegetative growth upward along the vertical axis of the world, as well as the vibrant reproductive fertility of animal life. His headdress or horned head connects him with horned male animals that represent animal virility, plus the horns reflect the lunar crescent that also curves to tapered tips.

With the flow and flower of related cultures through the ancient world, phallic and horned gods related to Pançika/the Mountain God or Shiva, such as Osiris of Egypt, Pan, Dionysus, Cernunnos, Herne, Cruachan, and Freyr in Europe, spread and flourished in various regions.

The phallic significance for you: Walk through woodlands and growing greenery; sense deep within your cells your connection with the living things. Feel the rising, vital energy of Lord Pançika within you. Ponder his connection with the Mountain God/Osiris/Pan and other horned gods. Is there really any important difference?

Masturbate in the forest to feel this. Sense your deepest and highest connection with Nature throughout your body, and through the direct link generated by your phallus in particular. Masturbate in the light of the Moon during its various phases. Admire the sharp horns of the crescent; appreciate the rounded forms of gibbous and full phases that resemble the head of your penis in shape. Remember that with the Full Moon everything becomes expressed and visible; with the New Moon anything is possible!

Feel your connection with what the Welsh poet Dylan Thomas called "The force that through the green fuse drives the flower."

From the Indus Valley and Egypt

Though the details are lost in the murky haze of the millennia that separate our "present" from then, clearly the ancient civilizations of the Indus Valley and the Egyptians had contact and traded influences, as well as material goods. The connections, perhaps overland through the Middle East and also directly across the Red Sea, or down through the Indian Ocean as well, occurred extremely early.

Possibly the Indus Valley culture started (circa. 3300 BCE) slightly before Egyptian civilization (circa. 3150 BCE), however this is purely a matter of definitions and interpretations of evidence. Regardless of such details, the two great civilizations arose pretty much in synch, not only in terms of time frames, but also with many basic similarities of specific imagery and cultural content.

In fact, along the overland routes where doubtless at least some of the traffic between them passed, the Sumerian civilization had been flourishing in the Fertile Crescent (Eden?) since around 5000 BCE. That is where history as defined by the appearance of written records began, as far as we know.

The Sumerians however, had a different mind-set from the later Indus and Egyptian cultures. In Sumer, the gods were feared, offerings were intended to appease them, and people lived in dread of their divine wrath. Both the Indus people and Egyptians lived in river valleys as fertile as the Sumerians, though in far more secure locations with less concern over aggressive invaders.

Ancient Sumer was pretty much surrounded by access on land, amid hostile neighbors who later became people with their own kingdoms, such as the Hittites, Akkadians and Mitannis. Those neighbors looked upon Sumer, with its riches of agriculture, husbandry and other natural resources where the Tigris and Euphrates rivers converged, with envy. Thus the Sumerians were often forced to defend their turf.

The Indus Valley rivers and the Nile both produced tremendous abundance with their annual floods that brought rich silt from upstream. Their heartlands were easily accessible only from the river mouths of the deltas that connected them with the oceans. Inland, both river valley regions were naturally quite well protected from invasion, and enjoyed plenty of other resources as well as agricultural fertility.

Both of these cultures developed a far more secure, relaxed and celebratory attitude toward the Gods who began as personified forces of the natural environment and evolved over time into more humanized divine principles. Both viewed their Gods and Nature as a sort of extended family they were part of. They also had a lot more in common than this happy relationship with their deities: Sacred Serpents, the Sacred Bull and Cow, a Great Mother, a Phallic Father, the Holy Family, the Holy Child, Gods of Sun and Moon and Stars, plus Animal Gods. Other aspects of the two cultures also reveal similarities.

Apparently the Indus Valley people, like the Egyptians, actually made no distinction between the sacred and the secular; the spiritual and material worlds were seen as merely aspects of a single, divine reality. Likewise, the Indus Mountain God and Lord Osiris, the major phallic god the Egyptians, while not identical, clearly share a common ancestor in human experience of the essential qualities of males.

That common ancestor is the actual, sacred experience of male arousal.

For your purpose of remembering the phallic wisdom encoded in your cells, these phallic gods from these two cultures are a good place to start.

In Egypt, Menu (or Min) is the oldest form of the phallic god—a primordial Sky Father and Rain God. The veneration of Menu is among the most ancient prehistoric roots of Egyptian culture, and the practice continued throughout history with the annual Valley Festival. A standing, kingly figure with one arm raised to shoulder-level, the forearm vertical, Menu displays a full erection and his other hand holds the base of his penis. During the annual Valley Festival his ithyphallic figure was carried through the fields.

Menu is a humanized connection with the power of vegetative growth and regeneration. Menu also embodies the phallic power attributed to the early kings and later pharaohs of Egypt. He assures their personal sexual potency, as well as the abundant yields of the fields, which are considered one and the same. Menu is also a Moon God, associated with lunar cycles, a traditional phallic quality.

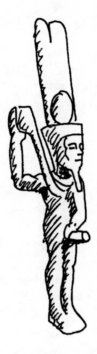

Menu, the Valley God of Egypt

It is said that the goddess and her husband simply came walking into Egypt, and brought civilization with them. Possibly this represents the arrival from the Indus culture of early forms of the Daughter of the Mountains and her husband, the Mountain God.

The phallic significance for you: Deep in your cellular awareness the reality of the phallic god abides—not a supernatural or religious being, rather an extremely powerful, empowering, and potent aspect of you that may be invited to emerge into full flower. This is neither the Mountain God, nor Osiris, nor any one of the many other forms of the phallic god, rather it's an actual innate aspect of your male humanity.

Such deities may be allowed to inspire this emergence into conscious awareness, however the phallic god within you is a direct, living experience of arousal and erotic ecstasy that connects you directly with all of the male ancestors within you and with the Divine, Nature, Gaia, or whatever you wish to call the totality of Life itself.

Nefertum: The Beautiful Young Lord of Morning

This is one of the oldest and simplest Creation stories in the world, from Egypt, and it has echoes in the Indus Valley cultural heritage...

From the unseen and unknown below the surface of the watery Void where nothingness abides—full, rich and fertile with all potentials though nothing is yet expressed—something stirs in the depths. Similarly from below the surface of a pool, from its hidden roots a lotus bud pushes up on a slender green stalk until it reaches above the surface. A small, delicate green cone aims upward, perfectly balanced, as if seeking something, until the soft warm sunlight of the early morning touches it and the bud begins to open. Creation is as natural as any living process!

A great mystery is the manner in which the lotus flower and the Sun God both come into being at the same moment, as if they create one another out of necessity.

For this flower, that opens a glorious crown of delicate blue-violet petals the color of the cloudless sky, is actually a god called Nefertum. *Lord of Fragrances! Handsome Young Phallic God of the Morning Sun! The Complete On Who Creates Himself—by a sacred act of physically loving himself, by pleasuring himself.*

The Egyptian Blue Lotus is actually both the phallus of the god and it is the Creator himself. The god and his phallus are One.

As the petals open, from the golden, fragrant heart of Nefertum's flowering is born the radiant Sun God Ra. In that mystical unity of early morning creative male energy, Nefertum and Ra are One. This is the first morning of Creation, and hereafter every morning the Handsome Young Phallic God of the Morning Sun is reborn.

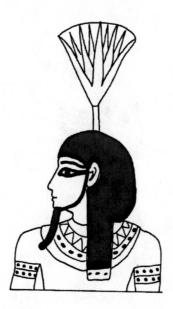

Neftertum, Lord of Fragrances

The phallic significance for you: As you learn Male Erotic Alchemy and transform and regenerate yourself, you reclaim the youthful virility and vibrant vitality of young manhood. Enjoy the special sweetness of those early morning erections that may bless you around daybreak. However entertaining and elaborate some of the following phallic myths are, this myth holds the essence of them all, enfolded into its petals.

Your penis grows like a lotus blossom and as it expands, you re-create yourself and your world. The head of your penis is the bud, and its blooming is the full-blooded, gloriously sensitive engorgement of your glans penis during arousal.

The Egyptian Blue Lotus is an actual plant. In fact it is a species of water lily called *Nymphaea careulea* that was used in Egypt as a sacramental substance, for it contains a mild euphoriant and aphrodisiac qualities that stimulate both men and women. You may wish to cultivate some of these water plants simply to enjoy the real thing and to masturbate in their presence in a meditative manner.

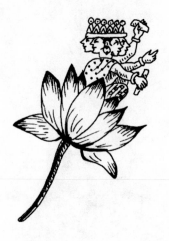

The Creator Brahma as Spirit of the Lotus

From the Indus Valley culture's later heritage come numberless images of the Creator Brahma seated upon a cosmic lotus. This equates the lotus with Creation itself, having a direct connection with the unseen Seed Source of All Things. In a deep sense this is a literal reality, in the same way that the stem of the lotus connects with its hidden root in the depths. The lotus is a symbol of Nature and the living essence of all things and beings in the Universe. This connects with the animistic view that everything is alive.

The Cosmic Holy Lingam of Creation

Return to the primordial Universe—newborn, bright and beautiful. Everything seems in perfect order so far, before any of the more complex stories have started to upset the balance. And yet to set things in motion, the balance must somehow be disrupted so that it can be restored. Thus two of the greatest gods begin to argue.

"*I AM the Creator,*" Lord Brahma insists, "*so of course, I was first! I made everything.*"

Vishnu smiles patiently. "*However, as the Sustainer, the credit for this Creation belongs to me. If I did not maintain and preserve it, nothing that appears would continue to exist.*"

"*What have you got to lose, if you admit that I was first, and that I created everything?*"

"*Beloved Creator, admit it: I AM the Supreme Lord!*"

"*No, no, beloved Brother, Sustainer though you are—*" and thus their pointless contending continues, quite politely in fact, yet it distracts them from the business of helping the Universe to unfold like the bud of a lotus, as it had been designed to do.

Suddenly a blazing white light appears, a pillar of blinding radiance that soars so high above and sinks so far below, that it appears truly limitless in extent!

"*Who are you?*" both Brahma and Vishnu cry out in astonishment.

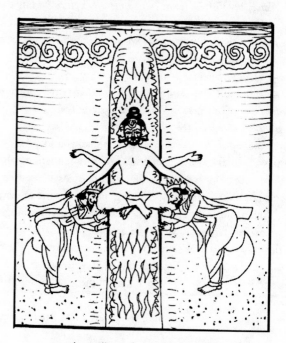

The Pillar of Limitless Light

"*I AM the One you both claim to be,*" *a mighty male voice speaks from the pillar of white light.* "*The Limitless Light of Love and Truth. I AM all of these: the Supreme Lord, Creator, Sustainer, and Regenerator, the Cosmic Lingam of the Auspicious One, Lord Shiva, I AM.*"

Brahma says, "*We are humbled, Great Lord!*"

"*Lord,*" *Vishnu says,* "*we both bow down before your omnipotent splendor!*"

Brahma says, "*However, we need to be absolutely sure that you are who and what you claim to be, before we can really surrender and totally honor you.*"

"*See for yourself,*" *the great voice replies mildly.*

So Brahma changes himself into a swan and flies upward beating snowy wings, to seek the top of the Cosmic Holy Lingam; Vishnu becomes a turtle with a horny shell and paddles downward, seeking the bottom of the radiant pillar.

Eventually the Brahma Swan enters a realm of celestial flowers that gently rain downward to broadcast the incredibly sweet fragrance of the Divine Nectar. Still, he finds no top to the Cosmic Shiva-lingam. Diving into the deepest depths of the abyss below, the Vishnu Turtle has no more success in finding a bottom to the radiant pillar.

When they return and meet one another again, Sustainer and Creator beg one another's forgiveness, and they fondly reconcile.

The voice of Shiva from the Cosmic Holy Lingam says, "*The truth is that all dualities, and even the Great Trinity of we Three Gods, exist only to remind us that in reality we are One. One in Three and Three in One.*"

The phallic significance for you: The creative, sustaining, and regenerative potency of your penis is far greater than you may have imagined. It has the power to take you deeper and higher than anything else in your embodied existence. Also, when you are totally, intensely aroused and in a state of mindfully alert attention to nothing but your erotic ecstasy, nothing else exists. There *is* no separate past, present, and future; nothing is greater or smaller, nearer or farther away, before or after. No separation exists. Your arousal is the only thing in existence and this is no illusion—it is truth.

This is the deepest and highest state that you can experience while embodied, and it provides you an actual taste of the great mystery of Oneness with All Things.

You can actually *feel* that nothing is separate from anything else.

The Heliopolitan Creation Story of Egypt

*B*efore anything happens, nothing exists except for the liquid chaos of a void called Nu. The swirling nothingness of Nu is not so much emptiness, as a flux of limitless possibilities, in which anything is possible, yet so far, nothing has yet happened.

Just as the receding waters after the annual high flood of the mighty Nile River subside and leave behind large mounds of fertile black soil washed downstream from the river's distant headwaters in Africa, a mound appears amid the nothingness of Nu.

This primordial mound is the first thing to appear from the nothingness.

Just as anything that persists in manifestation begins to acquire an identity, the mound continues to exist just long enough for some awareness to emerge: "I AM Atum," he tells himself, "I AM the Complete One: Lord of the Primordial Mound." Saying this in itself makes him more actual. With self-awareness he becomes a being.

His self-image grows more solid with each breath, with each beat of his heart, and he recognizes himself to have the ka, or sacred appearance, of a kingly man. He stands atop the mound that lifts like a small, dark island from the surrounding flux of Nu. He realizes that though he is complete, he stands alone.

Atum grows in awareness of himself, his form, his place, and his situation. "I AM, the Complete One, Atum," he says. "That I AM becoming. I AM the first and only thing in the midst of all this nothingness. However, unless I grow more solid and certain of my own existence, my own tangible reality, I could easily dissolve back into that fluid chaos of Nu from which I emerged. How can I make myself more real, more definite, happier and more balanced? To increase my confidence and awareness of myself will help me to continue my existence here!"

With both hands, Atum feels his own body, which begins to reassure him and increases his self-awareness. This also feels good, and he becomes aware of wonderful sensations from between his legs. His hands discover that tingling male organ of regeneration engorged with blood, standing stiff and asking to be touched.

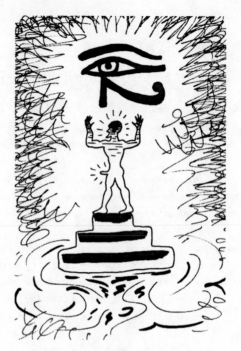

Lord of the Primordial Mound

As he begins to stroke his ultra-sensitive erection, the pleasurable sensations spread up his spine, and his heart opens like a lotus blossom in the growing light of a new morning. He continues to masturbate simply because he loves the sensations; his pleasure increases to bliss and then becomes ecstasy. The sensations climb to his head and fill his limbs. His entire body grows radiant with an indescribable glory.

"This is the best and most natural way to maintain my own happy, balanced existence as the Lord of the Primordial Mound, the Complete One, in the face of the chaotic forces of Nu that could sweep me away and dissolve my parts."

No one can say how long Atum continues his joyful masturbation standing upon the mound, before he approaches his first climax. Whatever the length of the measureless interval, eventually he can feel that something tremendously important and exciting is about to happen.

Somehow he knows that at this moment, he literally holds an infinite creative power in his hands. Gazing down upon the glory of the engorged phallus that he holds, he follows his instinct. Atum rolls onto his back, throws his legs up over his head, flexes his spine as far as he can and takes the head of his penis into his mouth. This feels so incredibly fine that it tips the scales.

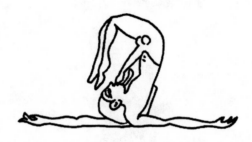

Atum's Autofellatio (Actual Egyptian graphic)

His ejaculation is powerful and copious. He nearly chokes on his own semen: he coughs twice, and expels from his lips the first god and goddess.

Shu, the Lord of Air, and his sister Tefnut, the Lady of Mist, appear.

With great wonderment and joy, Atum kneels and embraces his children, who already grow rapidly as young primordial gods do. "My beautiful son and daughter," he greets them, "you have emerged from my love for myself. I AM your father, Lord of the Primordial Mound, the Complete One, Atum, I AM.

"All that I want for you is your happiness and safety. So please take heed: stay away from the edge of the mound, or else you might be swept away into the void of Nu, from which this mound has emerged!"

Shu and Tefnut fondly embrace and kiss their father Atum, however being very young, like most children they are curious and love to explore their world. All too soon they disobey Atum; they go close to the edge of the mound, and they dip their toes into Nu. Nothing terrible happens, so they dive in for a swim. A wave of chaos surges and sweeps them away.

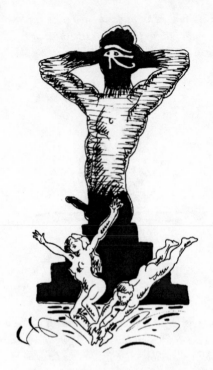

Lord Atum's disobedient Children

When Atum sees what has happened, he feels his heart shrivel in his chest, like a pinecone grown dry and brittle on the branch of a tree. "Oh, what can I do to find my children and bring them back to me safely?" He clutches his brow. "If I venture into Nu myself, most likely I'll be lost or dissolved, and the whole story will end!"

From his brow, his Wisdom Eye speaks, "Send me out like a ship sailing into Nu, and I will find your lost children and bring them back to you."

Atum brings his hand down from his brow, and the Wisdom Eye floats before him, like a ship made of glowing violet light. "Would you do that for me?"

"Of course," the Eye of Wisdom says, "only you must stay here and be safe."

"Thank you, I will remain."

So the Wisdom Eye of Atum sails off into the liquid chaos of Nu and vanishes from sight. The Lord of the Primordial Mound stays there and keeps himself balanced and happy by masturbating, though eventually he begins to forget about his children and the Eye. In fact, he replaces the Eye with two new ones, putting *in his face the Sun and the Moon to light the darkness of the void. His right eye is the Sun, and his left eye is the Moon.*

Eventually the Wisdom Eye reappears from Nu and brings Atum's children Shu and Tefnut safely back to him.

Atum receives them with open arms; he embraces them both and weeps for joy. His children, who have been lost and afraid, are every bit as happy to be reunited with their father. However in their familial joy, they all forget one thing.

The Wisdom Eye hovers nearby, feeling forgotten.

"Oh, there you are," Atum says, as he wipes his tears of joy and sees it. "No, I have not forgotten you, and I will never forget the wondrous thing you have done for me! This creation almost ended, but you have saved the day, so it may continue."

He beckons, and the Eye glides closer; it hovers above his open hands. "In order to thank you, and to always remember what you have done, let me give you a place of honor, above the new eyes that I put in my face."

So Atum places the Wisdom Eye back upon the middle of his brow and there it remains today.

Still the story of this creation is only beginning. The young gods Shu and Tefnut become the parents of the next generation. Their children are Geb the Lord of Earth, and Nut the Lady of Sky. Thus is established the Below and Above of this world.

As the Lord of Air, Shu realizes that this new son and daughter will probably repeat the same thing that their parents did and reproduce. He decides that perhaps the lineage would benefit from diversity. So Shu arranges the marriage of his daughter Nut to the primordial Sun God Ra.

However, as Geb, the Lord of Earth stretches below the Lady of Sky above him, he gazes upward at her beauty with longing and desire, and his penis grows erect. As the Sun God, Ra only can keep an eye upon his young bride in the daytime. During the daytime, the Lady of Sky wears the chaste blue garb of the faithful wife of Ra.

However, with each nightfall, Nut sheds that blue robe and became Nuit, the Lady of Stars, and the Queen of Infinite Space. In this form, she spreads her starry wings and descends upon her brother, Geb. He lies stretched out on his back, fully aroused, his phallus aimed upward and ready for her to mount him.

The Moon God, whose home is in the left side of the face of Atum, sees what is happening. He tells their father Shu, who goes immediately to where his children lie, coupled in their nightly bliss.

Instead of saying anything to them, Shu simply takes hold of his daughter Nut, in her starry form of Nuit, and with both arms raises her back up to her place high above.

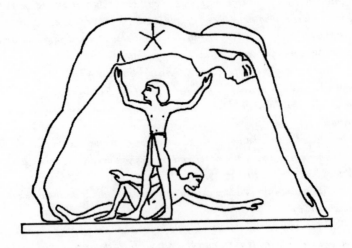

Shu separates Nut from Geb

His son Geb remains startled and stunned, his erection still vertical, only now it is revealed. That *revelation* inspires the Egyptian obelisk, the axis of the world that still connects the Below with the Above.

Though her father Shu, as Lord of Air, keeps his daughter the Sky in place above her brother the Earth below, as happens with primal deities, she has already conceived multiple offspring.

Her children are the generations of the Great Gods of Egypt and their children.

Still, as the root cause of all this burgeoning diversity, the family tree of the Egyptian Gods, the God of Origin, Atum persists.

The Lord of the Primordial Mound, the Complete One stands to this day, pleasuring himself in order to maintain the integrity and the forms of the whole of Creation that emerges from his self-love. His ecstasy sustains the structural unity of deities, human beings, and the Universe as a whole.

His constant self-pleasure keeps his Wisdom Eye open and thus he watches over all and maintains the cosmic order of everything.

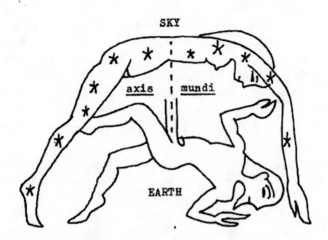

The Phallus of Geb as the World Axis

The phallic significance for you: Always remember that your penis, its arousal, pleasurable stimulation and ecstatic sensations, are a vibrant, living echo of your own origins: literally. Regardless of your actual relationship with your biological father, good, indifferent or not so good, you came into existence through his erection and ejaculation.

Your heritage as an embodied human male with this divine phallic potential derives primarily from your deepest ancestry. Your own creation is part of the ongoing processes that create the entire world and the Universe in which you find yourself. The ongoing creation of the world you live in is identical with your self-creative process.

As you pleasure yourself, remember that these ecstatic sensations express your male creative energy; and your ecstasy creates, sustains and regenerates you with life, wisdom and strength.

The Naked Saints

Another major religion aside from Hinduism emerged from the ancient Indus Valley civilization: the heritage of the Jains, or the Victorious

Saints. Less well known in the Western World than Hinduism and Buddhism, the Jains have an ancient culture and religion whose teachings share a common ancestry with many aspects of Hinduism and Buddhism.

The Jains practice a highly ethical path that includes extreme reverence for all living things. Non-violence is a central doctrine of their belief system. Its long history includes the lifetimes of twenty-four great teachers they call the *Tirthankara* or Propagators, considered pure souls. The word here paraphrased as "Propagator" also means literally, a "ford-builder" and refers to someone who helps others to cross a great, flowing river, from the other side to this side.

Jainism basically teaches that not only people and creatures have souls—everything has a soul. Non-violence is taken to an extreme in order to avoid causing harm and suffering to any living thing.

The first of the Propagators, a man called Most Excellent, is traditionally credited with bringing all the basics of civilization to his people, just as Osiris did for his people far to the west in Egypt. Most Excellent appeared at the end of the Stone Age just as people began to develop agriculture, husbandry and settled communities.

Most Excellent, like the subsequent Propagators who developed his teachings, is generally depicted naked, longhaired and often shown in a cross-legged meditative pose. This nakedness indicates purity of being, a naturalness and lack of ego-based identity. There is nothing lascivious about such nudity, on the contrary the Victorious Saints' teachings include the value of celibacy, or to refrain from sexual intercourse for the sake of social harmony.

Virtually every culture or religion that survives today has eventually developed some kind of codes to govern or control sexual behavior. The original intention was to preserve individual integrity and social harmony. This can be accomplished far more effectively when it comes from within the individual as a result of increased awareness, along with informed and empowered choice.

Even Far Eastern religions are often prone to repressive and prudish attitudes concerning sexual behavior. Some contemporary devotees claim that the Shiva-lingam does not actually represent the penis of Shiva, that it is a purely abstract symbol of a lofty abstract principle. However Shiva himself makes plain in the *Linga Purana* that this is not so as he says: "Every time there is an erection, human or animal, I AM present."

More important here is the fascinating common ground of the nature of the Propagators and the broader East Indian concept of sadhus or holy men. The Propagators and Lord Shiva clearly share similar origins and a parallel nature of extreme asceticism from early on, plus both stem directly from the Indus Valley culture. In practice, such men renounce all worldly attachments, even garments, and fearlessly trust Nature and the Universe to provide their needs as they seek to live in union with the Divine.

Today the Hindu holy men called Naga Babas still live naked and without belongings. They sometimes migrate annually between northern and southern locations, or live in the forests and mountains as the naked holy men of the Victorious Saints still do at times, and as the Mountain God Lord Shiva himself did.

Naga Baba literally means a naked or sky-clad father, uncle or grandfather, who does not shave his face and wears his hair in thick, unshorn locks. Many, though not all, Naga Babas are Shiva devotees, and they may carry the trident Shiva is depicted with. Such men have chosen a radical separation from mainstream culture for spiritual purposes, and make a total commitment to liberation from worldly illusions.

Though living naked, such holy men to this day often smear their skin with ashes. This indicates that such a man is dead to himself, as the ash is a reminder of fleeting human life—the mortality so evident on the cremation grounds. This is not necessarily a rejection of the past, so much as the indication of a new stage of awareness beyond individual limitations.

Such nakedness can also be understood as a return to closer connection with the natural Divine Self. After a lifetime of experience, the man prepares for his richest rewards of spiritual evolution by the reunion with his essence. All distracting, limiting and unnecessary possessions, accessories, and practices are left behind as he confronts the cosmos directly.

Even Lord Shiva, the Auspicious One, who began as the Mountain God and Lord of Yogis, may have a one time been an actual human holy man born sometime in the last five to seven thousand years. If so, most likely his practice of Tantrick Arts and semen retention, his choice not to ejaculate when he made love or masturbated, helped to turn him into a phallic god.

Male Erotic Alchemy can definitely do something of the kind for *you!*

The phallic significance for you: Having lived a full and long lifetime of experience, responsibility and learning, imagine that you are given the chance to return into Paradise while still living in your body! As you return to the pure state of Original Innocence, will you need your clothing? Or would it only serve as a reminder of who you really are not, the limited personal and egoic self?

None of those aspects of the conditioned ego that identifies with various belongings and social roles are really who you are in your deepest and highest essence. The implication is, "Why trust a divine expression that insists on wearing clothing?"

Claim your own significance for nakedness as a spiritual experience, without reference to any particular culture or religion. It's simply natural and honest.

CHAPTER THREE:

RENUNCIATION AND THE RETURN TO PLEASURE

The Mountain God at the Forest Hermitage

In a great forest lives a small community of hermits practicing the most challenging austerities and fire sacrifices. At this hermitage reside many great scholars and wise holy men along with their wives. However much of their attention has become occupied with matters of ritual, such as the precise manner of performing the fire sacrifices, and the cleansing rituals of virtuous bathing, how to eat reverently, marathon chanting and prolonged meditations.

In the role of a mendicant, Shiva the Mountain God and Lord of Yogis, wanders the woodlands naked, fasting, meditating all the time and performing the strictest austerities. These practices have bestowed upon him special abilities, plus he even manifests siddhis, or miraculous powers over the material plane. He has no possessions, though a tiger of the forest has deeded to him its skin. The devoted creature has volunteered to become a rug, asking that when it dies naturally it should be skinned and its hide tanned for Shiva's use.

Shiva also haunts cemeteries and the crematoriums along the riversides where the dead are burned upon pyres. He smears himself with ashes from the pyres in order to keep himself mindful of human mortality, as well as for protection from the abundant insects of the forests and river valleys. So in this role of a mendicant, to beg for his food, he approaches the saintly hermits of this particular forest retreat.

He arrives at their gate holding in both hands a human skull, while his penis stands at full erection from between his thighs, a combination of attributes that has a most curious influence upon his hosts and their family members.

They see an incredibly beautiful young man, naked and with uncut hair bound up in a topknot, his elegant mustaches and beard unshaven, handsome and strong, he is smeared with ash from head-to-toes. His aura radiates the vivid rays of his spiritual power; an uncanny light flickers from his eyes. This young holy man exerts an almost irresistible attraction to both the male hermits, and also to their virtuous wives.

To the dismay of the sages, their usually dignified wives and daughters rush out upon sight of the dazzling visitor immediately after his arrival within the compound. The women run to Shiva with offerings, they toss garlands of fragrant flowers around his neck, and hold bowls of ripe, luscious fruit before his face. The women lose all their customary social graces and restraint, as they cluster around the young man, like fish swarming to a handful of breadcrumbs thrown onto the surface of a pool. They take hold of his hands, and plead for him to attend them, to come with them.

As he stands among them with a slight smile, yet unresponsive to their entreaties and grasping hands, the women begin to divest themselves of their jewelry. They throw away their finger rings, nose rings, earrings, bracelets, necklaces and ankle bangles. They unbind their hair, unwind their garments from their bodies, and surround him as an encircling group of naked, pleading and giggling women.

At first the group of hermits simply stands at a distance, frozen and open-mouthed in disbelief. They have spent many years, sometimes a long lifetime of challenging austerities and rituals, and yet they have not attained special powers, which the remarkable aura of Shiva makes obvious that he possesses!

The oldest sage, their leader by default, steps forward: "What is your name?" he demands.

Shiva greets this demand with silent bemusement, only a slight smile appears upon his exquisite face. This lack of response, along with their insane jealousy infuriates the holy men, who converge as a mob. They fling aside their women and seize Shiva. As some hold him captive—though in fact he does not resist— one among them lunges forward with a knife and cuts off his erect penis.

Shiva does not react visibly to this terrible mutilation, any more than he did to the desperate lust of the women, the leader's question, or the many male hands that hold him fast. Rather, he simply regards them calmly, still smiling slightly, and then closes his two eyes. At that moment the vertical third eyelid upon the middle of his brow opens and a brilliant light shines forth from his Third Eye. Then he opens the first two so that all three eyes are open wide.

*When the horrified assailant drops the severed male organ of Shiva to the
ground, it lands upright, and immediately expands to enormous proportions, to
connect the Earth with the Sky.*

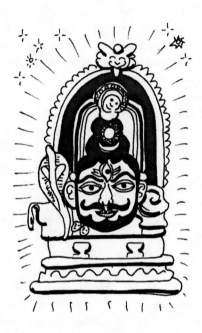

The Shiva-lingam of Light

*"My goodness," cries the oldest hermit, their leader, "this young yogi is
actually a mighty god! He must be one of the major deities, come to us in human
form, to test our ability to recognize him! The only effective penance we can do
now is to honor this Holy Lingam."*

Thus the veneration of the male organ of Shiva comes into being.

*As the sages begin to worship the Holy Lingam, their virtuous women regain
their composure and modesty, and remember their roles as wives and mothers and
daughters to the men.*

*"In this manner," Shiva tells them, "you have learned the limitations of
reason and propriety. Rapturous abandon is a more natural and powerful path
to the Divine than is denial and celibacy. Experience the mystical bliss in which*

the Lover and the Beloved are One, in which the separate sense of self dissolves in Oneness with the Great Supreme Self. You do not need to perform this Holy Lingam ritual with any other partner but the Supreme Self. Thus the droplet of ecstatic nectar returns to the Ocean of Bliss that is its origin, the reality of Oneness. Forget yourself to remember your own Divine Nature."

While the inhabitants of the hermitage institute these new practices to honor the Holy Lingam and engage in the Tantric Arts of Love, Shiva remains among them for a short while. They discover that in fact, the violent act has not actually been able to mutilate Shiva's divine form. He remains whole after all—that awful episode only allowed him to teach them.

He also teaches them the virtues of his favorite beverage, bhang, as a divine elixir. "As Soma is the drink for the Gods," he says, "this bhang provides mortal humans with a pleasurable experience of mystical rapture that will always remind you of my presence, even when I am gone from among you. In this rapture you will forget your conscious, limited human self and in ecstatic trance discover your spiritual nature as an incarnation of the Divine. Use it wisely."

Shiva squats in the yard, to grind the potent hemp with a huge mortar and pestle braced between his legs. He instructs the hermits in how to brew a refreshing elixir of the fragrant and intoxicating herb. Then he picks up again the human skull that he often carries on his wanderings.

As he promised, after he leaves them, whenever the hermits drink the bhang, with blissful attention focused upon the Shiva-lingam, they still feel the presence among them of Shiva, the Lord of Yogis, and the Lord of the Dance, the Auspicious One.

The phallic significance for you: Never imagine that your penis is anything less than an expression of the Divine Phallus, the axis of the world than connects Earth with Sky, and Below with Above. Remember that denial of the holiness of the body, and strict austerities will not connect you with the Source of All Things as effectively as to practice the arts of erotic ecstasy with purity of heart and noble purpose.

Keep in mind that the lessons of pain and suffering become repetitive and limiting over time, while the conscious deliberate practices of pleasure and ecstasy open the doors of perception to limitless possibilities.

If you choose to employ hemp in a sacred and sacramental manner as part of your spiritual practice, do so moderately, responsibly and wisely in a manner that enhances your awareness and appreciation for your body, its potentials, and the unfoldment of your life. In this book, the use of hemp is neither advocated nor condemned, but honored as an individual choice.

Daughter of the Mountains Claims the Lord of Yogis

Shiva has for measureless times defended the heavenly abode of the Gods from the evil Demons of the Netherworld that constantly seek to invade and take their celestial home from the Gods, in order to live there themselves. Only the greatest of divine warriors, Shiva with his trident, his drum of war, and his conch to sound his victories, has successfully defended that realm for eons.

However, Shiva has fallen in love with a mortal woman, and when inevitably she dies, in his grief he retires from defending Heaven into a cave on the side of Mount Kailash. There he leaves behind all worldly pleasures to study the scriptures and to meditate. Meanwhile those pesky Demons invade yet again; this time they manage to drive the Gods from their heavenly palaces.

The Great Divine Mother—who like Isis, her Egyptian equivalent, is the Living Soul or animating force of the Universe, bringer of skill, love, potency and wisdom—sees with great concern what has happened. On a high spiritual level, she is the life-force energy of Lord Shiva, activated by the ongoing spiritual union of his Holy Lingam with her universal expression as the Cosmic Womb. However, in the material world of duality and diversity she has never actually met him in person.

Shiva has grown immeasurably in his spiritual powers, among them his detachment from cause and effect, good and evil, and all dualities. In his state of Oneness with All Things, he thus remains unconcerned that the Demons have conquered Heaven and driven out the gods.

The Gods approach The Great Divine Mother for her help. "Please intercede with Shiva and ask him to help us!" they plead.

"You know that Shiva will no longer fight for you," she responds. "He has evolved too far above and beyond such dualistic concerns."

"So what can we do, Great Divine Mother?"

"Only a Son of Shiva will be able to drive the Netherworld Demons out, so that you can return to your proper place in the cosmic order. However, Shiva is so aware of the nature of suffering in the world, he refuses to engender any children, for that would cause more suffering."

"Is there anything you can do?"

The Great Divine Mother promises, "I will do my best."

Thus she takes birth as a lovely maiden named Daughter of the Mountains, the first child of the Holy Himalayas. Daughter of the Mountains goes to the cave where Shiva performs the strictest austerities of a solitary hermit. Upon sight of him seated cross-legged on a tiger-skin, naked with his three eyes closed, she instantly falls in love.

Daily she visits his cave to sweep the floor, and to scatter fragrant blossoms there, to seek his attention and favor. The gloriously beautiful and infinitely aloof hermit of Mount Kailash treats her with absolute kindness and gentle politeness—and also strict indifference. He already has one devotee, who acts as a manservant to do for him what his Lord is too withdrawn and unworldly to be concerned about.

Daughter of the Mountains hatches a plot, and makes the manservant promise to guard Shiva's sleeping pallet so that he will definitely remain chaste and not be bothered by visitors who might be attracted sexually to his beauty. Feeling that his chastity is protected until she herself has a chance to seduce him, Daughter of the Mountains departs into the rugged ranges to perform her own austerities. She seeks the equivalent for herself of the powers that he has attained.

Meanwhile a demon has spied upon her while she spoke with Shiva's manservant, so after she has been gone for a while, the demon uses its powers and transforms itself into a perfect image of Daughter of the Mountains.

Except that the demon has lined its vagina with deadly nails.

Though the manservant is fooled as well and Shiva receives the false Daughter of the Mountains just as graciously and with the same detachment he has always extended to the real Daughter of the Mountains, this one fools even him. Or perhaps he merely allows it to enter and believe it has succeeded in seducing him.

"She" flirts and dances for him while she undresses. His eyes open and he watches her. At last with a slight roll of his eyes, he beckons her. When the disguised demon mounts his lap to perform a sacred yab-yum of Tantric copulation with him, as his erection begins to penetrate the vagina lined with nails, he turns his penis into a sword.

The demon impales itself and dies. When Daughter of the Mountains hears of this, she flies into a rage, turns herself into a lion and races to the cave, where her glance of anger turns the manservant into a stone statue. Still, rather than proceed into the inner cave where Shiva is, she returns to the forest where she has been living.

There she lives naked, she fasts and she meditates all the time. Soon her abilities increase manyfold and she develops yogic powers and siddhis similar to Shiva's. The energy around her becomes so powerful, that it attracts the attention of Brahma the Creator, who looks upon her with wonder and favor.

"What can I do for you, my lovely child?" Brahma says kindly.

"I've done all I can to attract the love of the Mountain God," she replies, "and I've even taken a path like his. I've become a solitary hermit; I've done extreme austerities and attained some powers. Still, he remains aloof, and as you know, the Gods are still exiled from their heavenly homes, where the vile race of Demons has taken possession."

"Tell me whatever you want, and I will grant it."

"Perhaps it is my dark skin, Lord Father of Creation! Can you change my dark skin into a beautiful golden color like honey that glows in the sunlight of happiness?"

"Granted," the Creator says and smiles. "Only I'll have to split you in two to do this properly, so there will be a darker version of you and a lighter one."

"Whatever it takes," she says, without really considering the full consequences.

So Lord Brahma raises his hands in blessing and makes it so: the dark half of Daughter of the Mountains becomes She Who Destroys, the fearsome Mother of Time and Transformation called Kali, who cuts off the heads of men to awaken them spiritually from their illusions.

The brighter half of Daughter of the Mountains now has skin so luminous it shines like golden sunlight.

Shiva awakes from his self-induced trance of indifference upon sight of the newly radiant Daughter of the Mountains. "You are just the kind of perfectly beautiful and virtuous woman I would like to marry someday," he says.

"Therefore," she says, "you might as well marry me now!"

The phallic significance for you: Sadness and grief can throw you off from the path of your life. However, if you follow through and process these strong emotions, they may also lead you back to your true purpose. In retrospect you may even reclaim not only your joy, but also a new stage of even greater purpose and fulfillment.

Just as Shiva withdrew from involvement following the death of his mortal lover, sometimes you need to give yourself a break from relationships. This is a great time to refocus on yourself and to refine your skills of self-pleasure and to cultivate erotic energy without ejaculating often.

When you work on yourself and keep your focus to become more self-sufficient than ever in reclaiming your happiness, this eventually changes your aura and makes you more attractive than ever to just the right person or persons. Trust the process.

The First and Foremost Son of Shiva: Ganesh

*A*s he used to do before his marriage, the Lord of Yogis still often withdraws into the solitude of his cave to meditate, or he wanders in the Phallic Forest Primeval, naked and alone.

He offers Daughter of the Mountains, in what she takes as an insult, a rag-doll and tells her to hold and cuddle it instead of seeking to have a baby of her own. "I will not let my husband's absence get in my way," she decides. So Daughter of the Mountains rubs unguent oil into her thigh, scrapes off the resulting film, rolls it into a mass and molds it into her child. Thus she immaculately conceives her son and brings him to life as she breathes her own powers into him.

He is a beautiful young man every bit as handsome, strong and virile as Shiva.

Daughter of the Mountains names her new child and companion Ganesh, "Remover of Obstacles, and Lord of New Beginnings." She educates him to act as a scribe, teaches him everything she knows, and assigns him as the guard of her own bedchamber door to keep out strangers who might be attracted to her irresistible beauty and try to seek her favors. Thus he is also called "Guardian of the Threshold."

Meanwhile her husband meditates and it comes to him that perhaps he should not be so neglectful of his beloved wife, so with the intention to apologize, he returns. He has no idea who the new guard at her threshold is. When Ganesh—similarly unaware of who the handsome naked yogi is—bars his way, Shiva flies into a rage and beheads the young man.

Daughter of the Mountains rushes forth from her chamber. When she sees what has happened, she screams, and backs away from Shiva. "Until you fix this, and give him a new head," she says, "I refuse to see you again!"

The Mountain God bows deeply. "My humblest apologies, beloved wife."

The original head of Ganesh had already rolled away across the floor and down the mountainside where a tiger ate it. So Shiva sends his followers out, to look for a new head. They return eventually with the beautiful head of a baby elephant, which Shiva successfully attaches to the decapitated, yet living body of Ganesh.

In this manner the Lord of Yogis and his wife Daughter of the Mountains, with their child Ganesh become a happy family. Though Shiva is his stepfather, the two become as close as an actual son and father can be, despite their unfortunate first introduction.

Finally, as they live together in harmony, Daughter of the Mountains encourages Shiva to accept worldly pleasures as part of his spiritual path. She thaws his detached heart with her warmth and pure-hearted sensuality.

Ganesh is given the titles of Guardian of the Threshold, Patron of New Beginnings, and Remover of Obstacles to Happiness. The Mountain God adds patronage of the arts to his own repertoire of concerns, and the sympathetic nature of Daughter of the Mountains also stirs his concern for suffering in the world.

His stepson, whose elephant trunk suggests a flexible and prehensile phallus, has a gentler, more approachable and appealing quality than his sometimes stern and intimidating foster-father. Shiva still haunts the cremation grounds and cemeteries at times, to meditate upon mortality and the grief of survivors. He gives Ganesh one of the graveyard rats—a symbol of wisdom—to ride upon.

This new stepson becomes the leader of Shiva's spiritual army of followers, sometimes seen as Nature Spirits, which is why Ganesh is also called Lord of Hosts.

The Mountain God's supreme symbol, however, remains the Shiva-lingam, the image of his phallus, which is also the axis of the world.

The phallic significance for you: Each member of this Holy Family is an aspect of you. The Mountain God is you as the phallic god that relates your human form with the universal design and purpose. Daughter of the Mountains is your social relationship with others, which may include family and extend to others beyond that immediate circle. Ganesh embodies possibilities that come from both of his parents, his actual mother and his stepfather. His stepfather's phallic energy is intense and cosmic; Ganesh is more warm-hearted and approachable.

Though the erotic energy generated by your phallus may be cultivated most effectively in solitude or in phallic brotherhood with a partner or partners, the energy itself does not exist in isolation, rather it connects through your heart and mind into all of your relationships.

Shiva's Second Son: Skanda

*D*aughter of the Mountains' consistent and pure-hearted adoration, plus her powers as the Great Divine Mother, the Soul of the Universe, has won over the heart of Shiva. During their prolonged and sacred Tantric lovemaking the dualistic nature of manifestation collapses back into the Oneness of Source. Shiva practices semen retention, meaning that he does not ejaculate, instead he keeps the erotic energy in his body; he does this for two reasons, to cultivate ever-higher erotic energy, and also to avoid conceiving a child that he feels will only add to the suffering in the world.

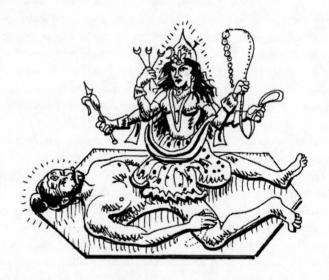

Divine Consciousness and Cosmic Energy Encoupled

However his new bride has her own agenda. She feels a strong maternal instinct to conceive a child by her husband. As Shiva's erotic energy circulates down the front of his body and back up his spine, this generates the Divine Nectar within his brain so that his head begins to emanate a rainbow nimbus. The Lady takes a small piece of Shiva's aura from the crown of his head within the topknot of his hair, a rainbow seed of his spiritual essence.

This bit of a rainbow she sends to the exiled Gods, who bestow it upon the river goddess named Ganga. Ganga cools the radiant rainbow seed in her icy waters until it forms a Mountain God seed. This seed she takes in her hands and reverently carries it to the Phallic Forest Primeval, where she plants it with devotion in the fertile detritus of the forest floor. In this place, anything planted will grow.

From the seed sprouts a virile new, young form of Shiva, named Skanda. This beautiful young god named Skanda, who is also a lover of his fellow men, raises a great army of followers, storms the heavenly realm, drives out the Demons, and restores the Gods to their rightful homes. The Macedonian conqueror Alexander the Great is also said to be an incarnation of Skanda.

Now, Daughter of the Mountains has managed to live up to her promise to the Gods. She is also transformed from a swarthy maiden to a golden goddess with the radiance of sunshine, plus her scheming has brought about the birth of the new young phallic god Skanda. He becomes the god of conflict resolution, the patron of male homosexuals, and the guardian of the gates of the heavenly realm.

However the one thing she has not succeeded in is to win the full-time husbandly devotion of Shiva. Plus she feels the strong urge many married women do to become a mother herself, however the God of Mount Kailash refuses. Though he is happy to engage in limitless amounts of Tantric coupling with her, for they embody the dynamic of plus (+) and minus (−) polarities in the cosmic order, Shiva tells her all along that to conceive a child of his loins would only add suffering to the world.

There is another version of the origins of Skanda:

Long, long ages in the past, after the Mountain God has become the Lord of Yogis, he practices semen retention, that is regardless of whether or not he engages in erotic activity, he controls himself from ejaculating.

Of course because of who he is, Shiva's seed will always create something or conceive a child on those rare occasions when he spills it.

In order to continue to develop his Tantric practice, Shiva allows Agni, the God of Fire, to perform fellatio upon him for prolonged periods, and it becomes a contest between his own erotic self-regulation and the ability of the God of Fire to perform exquisite oral stimulation of Shiva's sacred phallus.

Finally, in this case Agni triumphs, or Shiva simply decides to surrender to the ejaculatory orgasm he so seldom experiences. His seed spurts heroically into *the God of Fire's mouth and is swallowed. Immediately in the God of Fire's belly a child is conceived. As these are all deities, within moments Shiva's first son, Skanda is born from the God of Fire.*

Due to his conception by two male gods, the newborn godling becomes patron of male homosexuals and he is given the job of guarding the gates into the heavenly realm.

In his honor, the great sages of later times sometimes perform a fire sacrifice in which they ejaculate into their sacred fire.

The phallic significance for you: An important practice for human males is to learn to make ejaculation a choice, rather than something that simply happens when you lose control of the level of your arousal. At the same time, too much focus on control can be limiting to the spontaneity and mystery of existence. Still, choosing not to ejaculate during sustained, high quality arousal is a powerful tool of Male Erotic Alchemy.

The "Home of the Gods" on top of Mount Meru, the World Mountain represents the crown of your head. It stands atop the *Axis mundi* or World Axis. This macrocosmic axis corresponds with the microcosmic axis of your spine. Just as your spine has thirty-three vertebrae, there are said to be thirty-three Gods that live at the summit of Mount Meru. When you cultivate your erotic energy without ejaculation, the energy rises from the root at the base of your spine to the crown of your head. The Mountain God is your consciousness; his wife Daughter of the Mountains is your energy.

Recognize that none of the details of these mythic stories are merely abstract symbols; rather, they all represent aspects of your own body and your experience as a human animal in this world. In the later part of this book you will learn more about the value of cultivating your erotic energy as you would tend a garden for optimal growth and flowering, and you discover exactly how to accomplish this.

Ayyappa: The Third Son of Shiva

*A*nother crisis arises when the Demons steal the jar that contains the elixir upon which the extended lives of the Gods depends. Both the Gods and the Demons are actually beings called demi-gods, only long-lived rather than *truly immortal, unless they drink Divine Nectar, which can extend their lives indefinitely.*

The Moon God, who is able to transform ordinary pleasure into Divine Bliss, creates the Divine Nectar. Whenever he fills a jar with the elixir, he provides it to the Gods, who are willing to generously share some of it with the Demons. However it is well known that the Demons, should they possess the Divine Nectar would not share it but would keep it all for themselves. This is why the Moon God gives it to the Gods to be fairly shared among all the demi-gods.

On a certain occasion the Demons manage to steal the jar of Divine Nectar from the Moon God just as he is about to deliver it to the Gods. Vishnu the Lord Sustainer understands all possible strategies to maintain and preserve the creative processes of the Universe, so he employs a brilliant strategy.

On this occasion Vishnu assumes an exquisite female form called "Enchanted One." She appears as a classically gorgeous woman with fragrant jasmine blossoms in her hair. Enchanted One arrives mysteriously before the Demon stronghold, where she dances slowly along the front porch before the gates. The music of her ankle bells indeed enchants and enthralls any male heart, regardless of who he might be!

The Demon King and his followers, lustful creatures always avidly seeking the loveliest females, watch Enchanted One with huge eyes, and they fall totally under her spell. In this manner Vishnu distracts the Lord of Demons and his minions in order to retrieve the Divine Nectar. The Demons are blinded by lust—totally dazzled and entranced by Enchanted One. "She" has them wrapped around her little finger.

Enchanted One easily persuades the Demon King to allow her to dispense the Divine Nectar. "I'll be fair in how I distribute it," she says, "as none of you can be expected to be impartial, not even you, Great Lord!" The Demon King nods and smiles and hands over the jar.

Vishnu calls his Solar Eagle, who flies down and carries him back to the top of Mount Meru, where Vishnu returns the Divine Nectar to the Gods.

Shiva does not happen to be present when Vishnu in the female form of Enchanted One accomplishes this most beneficial and skillful act of deception to preserve the cosmic order.

However the Lord of Yogis hears of this charming exploit from a wandering sage who often visits the Lord and Lady of the Mountains. So with his wife, Daughter of the Mountains, Shiva goes to visit the Lord Sustainer.

He appears, holding his trident, smiling radiantly in his handsome, virile splendor. "I've witnessed your wondrous powers, O Sustainer. Only I have not seen the famous Enchanted One, your lovely female form, this latest strategy to keep universal balance and harmony in place. If the Demons had kept the Divine Nectar, they alone would have lived longer and the Gods would have aged and perished, like mortals. However, as always, you saved the day!"

Daughter of the Mountains smiles. "Yes, beloved and Supreme Lord Sustainer, and Dreamer of Universes, whose couch is the Cosmic Serpent!" She praises him sincerely, with both hands pressed together before her luscious breasts. "Please, Lord Vishnu, we are most curious to see this beautiful female aspect of you, that has saved the day! Grant us, we pray, this boon to see you as Enchanted One."

"Please," Shiva says, "I am most eager and curious to see her."

The Sustainer smiles serenely upon his honored visitors. "Oh best of the Gods, Shiva, Lord of the Mountain, how can I refuse you, who are part of me? After I returned the Divine Nectar to the Gods and they all drank of it, one of the Demons disguised himself as a God, and tried to also drink. The Sun God told me of this, just as he began to drink, so I threw my Divine Discus, which cut off his head. Only his head by itself became immortal!"

"Yes, that immortal head still flies around!" Shiva says. "I have seen it passing across the sky like a comet."

Again the Sustainer bestows a dreamy smile. "Now, because you have asked, I will show you this beautiful form I assumed, that arouses the desire of men, and which they value most highly." With these words, he vanishes from the sight of the Lord of the Mountains and his wife.

The divine couple remains where they are, looking all around them in every direction. Then Shiva spies a glorious garden, lush and green with many trees having red leaves and colorful flowers that bloom everywhere. Bees buzz and floral fragrances drift on the breeze... and there he sees a most exquisitely beautiful woman!

An enchanting woman stands playing with a ball. She tosses it into the air and throws it here and there. She chases it playfully and continues her play in the garden. She seems totally absorbed in the innocence of her game. Her bare breasts dance with her graceful motions, and then her shy gaze looks up, to meet Shiva's enraptured gaze directly.

Shiva totally forgets his entire entourage, plus the fact that his wife stands beside him. The lovely woman in the garden again tosses the ball, which bounces

*and rolls from sight. As she begins to follow it, on a gust of breeze the skirt that is
her only garment falls from her waist as she moves.*

Shiva's heart is full of nothing but her.

*He grows aroused and loses his mind. Oblivious to his companions, he rushes
forward into the garden, full of desire for her. He loses all common sense and
shame.*

*Naked as the breeze has rendered her, the woman acts shy and a bit evasive.
She flees his advancing steps and hides herself behind a tree, though she does not
stay there, aware that otherwise he will catch her immediately. Rather, she keeps
moving, and he follows her as persistently as a bull elephant follows an elephant
cow when they are in heat. He catches her in his arms, pulls her hair and holds
her body to his own, and thrusts his hips against her.*

She only laughs, like chiming bells, and pushes him away.

*As Enchanted One, the illusory female form created by Vishnu, escapes his
arms, Shiva spills his semen and runs after her, still fully aroused. Hi seed, which
cannot fail to create, continues to spill as he runs like a wild male elephant. At
each place the droplets fall, great golden Shiva-lingams spring up!*

*He continues to pursue Enchanted One over rivers, and lakes, and mountains,
forests and gardens, and where the great sages live, creating golden Holy Lingams
all the way along. At last he catches up with her and they make passionate love,
while Daughter of the Mountains watches from a distance, shocked and envious.*

*Then in the heat of passion Vishnu even reverts to his beautiful male form,
which has no effect upon the intense lovemaking of these two great deities. They
are so enthralled in their bliss that it does not matter that both lovers are male.*

*Finally, when Shiva is drained of all his semen, he comes to his senses and
realizes what had happened, how Vishnu's glamour as an all-attractive, alluring
woman, has enchanted him.*

*Shiva returns to Daughter of the Mountains, not sure what she will say.
His wife only smiles graciously and says, "With my Limitless Love for you and
my infinite understanding, you are completely forgiven for your indiscretion.
Hopefully you enjoyed yourself and learned something."*

"Thank you, my Beloved," her husband says humbly.

Then with their entourage they return home.

*Meanwhile Vishnu returns to his female form of Enchanted One and gives
birth to Shiva's third son, named Ayyappa, before he returns to his original male
form and resumes his place reclined on the Cosmic Serpent.*

When Shiva hears of this new birth, again he visits Vishnu who reclines upon the Cosmic Serpent and holds the new child on his lap.

"Only you," Shiva says to Vishnu, "could enchant me and make me lose my mind. Despite all of my austerities, desire overcame me, and it did not even matter when I realized that you had resumed your male form! I have learned that worldly pleasures serve the loftiest spiritual purposes, when we play in total innocence and purity of heart, and surrender to honest desire. My gratitude is boundless!"

The Lord Sustainer bestows upon the newborn child the gift of a necklace with a beautiful jewel. "Ayyappa will be called the son of two fathers and he combines our aspects, O Shiva. He will grow to become a mighty hero!"

Aware of the great destiny that awaits him, his divine parents leave the radiant infant on the banks of a river in a special place they have chosen for this purpose. The childless King of that country hears the infant's cries, finds him, and the glorious child instantly wins the King's heart. The King adopts Ayyappa as his own son, though shortly after this, the Queen gives birth to a son of his own flesh.

The King, however, considers Ayyappa his first-born and designates him as his royal heir.

The royal minister who envies the favor that the King bestows to Ayyappa, misleads the Queen, who feigns a fatal illness that her physician states can only be cured by drinking the milk of a tigress. The King despairs, aware of how close to impossible it is to obtain a tiger's milk without being killed.

However, brave and valiant Ayyappa volunteers, and marches off into the forest. Of course, because of his true parentage, Ayyappa is a powerful being. Some days later he returns to the court of the King, riding a tigress, followed by her cubs. This astonishing sight inspires the Queen to confess that the royal minister had misled her, and all of the conspirators beg forgiveness.

Ayyappa forgives everything, yet he declares that he must leave, and allow the actual son of the King's wife to be the crown prince. Ayyappa becomes a great hero, for he conquers Demons and inspires devotion to the Gods.

The phallic significance for you: In terms of your actual human male body, the Divine Nectar produced by the Moon God is the blissful biochemistry that you can generate when you cultivate erotic energy. It also refers to the Cowper's gland secretion, commonly called "precum" which may periodically emerge from the meatus at the tip of your aroused penis while you masturbate or engage in sexual activity.

While men vary individually in how much of this clear, slick fluid is produced, from nothing noticeable to quite a copious flow, more important is the quality of pure penile pleasure you experience during the kind of activity that may produce it. Remember that a phallic god often has lunar qualities, for the Moon is associated with the ultra-sensitive head of your penis.

The story also illustrates the fluidity of authentic male erotic attractions, for though the two major deities begin their flirtation in a male and female dyad, once the lovemaking becomes intense, a shift to a male couple makes no difference. Your sexuality is not important to the practice of Male Erotic Alchemy.

Whether women, other men, or both arouse you sexually, most important is your relationship with yourself. A man who purely loves his own penis is likely to appreciate and enjoy the penises and nakedness of his fellow men. This is natural and healthy.

When you trust the flow of events in your existence, relationships may be allowed to sort themselves out naturally, just as Ayyappa found his true purpose according to his actual origins. This is not about power over others, but about power from within you.

What the Three Sons of Shiva Mean

The three sons of Shiva relate to aspects of you and of every man. Ganesh is the aspect of you that may be mentored by someone powerful and become powerful in your own right, and in your own way. Skanda relates to the cultivation of your erotic energy, and appreciation for whatever bisexual or same-sex urges live somewhere within you. Ayyappa is your challenge to uncover who you really are in your innermost essence and to become only that authentic being.

Renunciation eventually makes you aware that to deny yourself pleasure is no more useful than unbridled self-indulgence. Authenticity arises from the balance between extremes. Because some suffering and pain is always a part of human existence, the conscious creation of pleasure serves to help reclaim this balance.

All three sons of Shiva depict your phallic inheritance from your forefathers, and suggest the benefits to you of both opening to a fluid and flexible sexuality, as well as learning to cultivate high erotic states while you retain your semen.

Chapter Four:

The Monotheistic Phallus

How did the belief in a single, omnipotent, invisible deity emerge from the numerous forms of animism, pantheism and polytheism of the ancient world?

For the Egyptians, like the East Indian cultures related to them early on, many varied and sometimes contradictory beliefs were available. No single orthodoxy or set of beliefs was consistently prescribed. Often it was an easy-going case of "Whatever works for you, is fine."

For example, one minor option in Egypt was a solar cult of the deity called *Aten*. The circle of the sun disk represented an invisible creator and bestower of life, as the architect of Nature and all living things, a divinity omnipresent, yet visible only through the myriad phenomena of the natural world. As such, the disk represented this giver of the gift, yet it was understood to be merely an abstract symbol of Aten.

Aten was the only deity worshiped by the famous King Akhenaten and his beautiful Queen Nefertiti, who were renegades in the context of 18th Dynasty Egypt.

Akhenaten and Nefertiti created their own spiritual community and banished the ancient gods from the Two Lands of Egypt. Yet they did not invent this belief in Aten from whole cloth. Such a variation on the Sun God had long existed in Egypt, centered at a place called *Annu*, or the City of the Sun.

The 18th Dynasty experiment did not last long, however it produced a legacy of exquisite art of unusual natural realism, plus it changed the world forever.

Heresy in Egypt

Though the Egyptians always remained highly phallocentric, meaning that the erect penis and the Male Mysteries were central to both religion and culture, among the ancient civilizations they alone never became truly patriarchal. Goddesses always shared equal importance with gods, as in nature both female and male animals are necessary for sexual reproduction and a balanced environment.

During the 18th Dynasty a most unique period helped to change the entire course of history thereafter. The brief revolutionary adventure of Akhenaten and Nefertiti who fostered an abstract, yet immediate, Nature-based monotheism evidently influenced the Semitic religions that arose not long after their heyday. Though his queen ruled with this king at least as his equal, it was the monotheistic aspect of their experiment that produced widespread and lasting repercussions.

Certain Semitic tribes of people spent time in Egypt during periods of famine, evidently more than once, before they returned to their homelands in what we now call the Middle East. Though no Egyptian inscriptions specifically mention these particular people by name, some later accounts of the Middle Eastern people describe their "enslavement" in Egypt.

In reality, no such institution as slavery of the kind common in the later Greco-Roman periods existed in Egypt. Though royalty might sometimes "own" groups of Nubian captives as personal servants and guards, the Egyptians did not generally practice ownership of people or forced labor, except in the case of convicted criminals who were sometimes compelled to work in gold mines.

Rather, due to the three seasons of the year as Egyptians viewed things, Flood, Growing, and Harvest, during the Flood season everyone who lived along the Nile shores was pretty much marooned and the fields were flooded. This prevented the peasants from working along the lower banks that were inundated. By cultural agreement, during this third of the year the general population helped to construct the sacred monuments for their Living God, the Pharaoh.

Not that all these workers were necessarily happy about it, however many of the devout Egyptians who did not separate the secular from the sacred in their minds, did this willingly. It was expected. Of course, some of those "foreigners" accepted into the Two Lands during times of famine elsewhere in the ancient world, may have viewed the whole experience quite differently.

It is true that Egypt usually experienced such abundance, with the fertile topsoil that washed downstream from the heart of Africa each year, the plentiful irrigation, and long hot growing season allowed two full crops, so immense surpluses existed. In fact, the ancients dug huge pits that they filled entirely with surplus grain.

Regardless of who "won," or who "wrote the history," as always we must read between the lines and look through the common assumptions of more recent beliefs in order to get a more accurate and clearer picture of the realities of ancient times.

Those Semitic peoples, some of whom later developed their own highly complex and successful traditions, originated from a region where—as in most of the Mediterranean world—the Great Mother goddess had long been venerated, accompanied by her consort, a Warrior God. She was considered the Mother of All Living, while he originally represented a strong virile male partner, to father her children and protect the group as leader of the warriors. Her supremacy would not last, however.

This balance of female and male deities began to shift towards male dominance over several thousand years with the spread of agriculture. Many people began to live in settled communities and even cities attached to cultivated lands. This urban lifestyle had an early heyday in the area embraced by the Tigris and Euphrates rivers.

Though later on three major monotheistic patriarchal religions sprang from these common roots, the earliest stories and characters have their origins in even older cultures such as Sumer, the Indus Valley, and Egypt. This Tigris and Euphrates region was geographically and culturally a major crossroads of the ancient world.

Plus, when considered with an open mind and clear eye, those earliest stories, whose repercussions remain strong in today's world, contain much that can be interpreted very differently from the way those three major religions now interpret them.

The Garden Story Revisited

The oldest cuneiform—the earliest known actual writing of Sumer—provides examples of the Garden Story with some thought-provoking variations quite different from the later versions.

For example, the Woman appeared or was created before the Man…

She is the first inhabitant of the Garden of Paradise, living naked and unashamed in Original Innocence. This Woman, by some accounts named Lilitu, has as a special friend and close companion, the wisest and most subtle creature of the Garden, though in these early days he walks upon two legs like a man: the Serpent.

The Serpent knows more about all the creatures, all the trees and flowers and green growing things of the Garden than any other being. The Woman learns all that she knows from this friend, for the Creator has blessed her and then left her there.

However, amid all that lush vegetation and among the harmonious creatures, even with the special friendship and company of the wise Serpent, she eventually realizes that she longs for something. She wants a companion of her own kind, only not a female like herself. The Serpent has shown her how all other creatures were created female and male so that they can propagate their own kind.

"Make for yourself that which you desire," the Serpent tells her.

"How can I do that?" she asks.

He explains the process.

Thus she takes her menstrual blood, mixes it with some clay and fashions herself a beautiful Man. She has seen the form of the Creator, who sometimes visits her in the Garden, so she bases the image upon his form. At the place on the body where it differs most from her own, she fashions a phallus in the image of her wise friend, the Serpent, to honor him.

Finished molding the figure, she kneels beside it, places her mouth over the clay mouth and breaths life into him. As the Serpent promised, he comes to life! At first the Man is amazed and delighted to live with this beautiful Woman.

However the Creator who brought the world forth from the Void announces: "She will become the mother of your children, and your wife."

"What does this mean?" Lilitu asks innocently, scratching her head.

The Man smiles sweetly, but his words sting her. "It means that you must bow down and worship me!"

"I bow to none but my great teacher, the Serpent," Lilitu says indignantly. "I am happy to co-exist with you as an equal partner, however, in reality I was here first. In fact, I created you! Yet I do not demand your subservience, only my own dignity and worth. I would like to be your friend and an equal partner."

The Man says, "Am I not created in the image of Our Father the Creator?"

"Yes, and yet it was I who created you..."

"Woman," the Creator says, "do as he asks, for indeed, you see how he is like a Living Image of myself. Am I not worthy of your worship?"

"You are worthy," Lilitu says. "And yet after you created me, you left me here in this place of beauty where the Serpent befriended me and taught me all I know. This Man, however, whom I myself created to be my companion, I will not bow down to."

"Then you must leave," the Man says. "I'll find another, better companion."

"Father Creator—" Lilitu begins to object.

"I am sorry, daughter," the Creator says, "however, it is not because of your disobedience to the Man that you must leave Paradise—you must leave because of your pride."

"This is wrong!" she cries. "Why should I not be proud of what I have learned and of my ability to create life? I have nothing to be ashamed of!"

However her protests do no good, for the Creator sends a messenger with a flaming sword to evict her, to force her out through the Gates of Paradise. Thus, out in the world beyond, Lilitu becomes a woman with the power of a goddess, who knows her own strength and always remembers her connection with the natural world.

Still in the Garden, the Man says, "Oh Father, will you not make me another female of my own kind who will serve me as my wife?"

"Be patient, child, for after you sleep next time, upon waking your prayers will be answered." Thus while the Man sleeps does the Creator fashion from a rib of his side another Woman.

It is this couple that the Creator warns about eating of the Fruit of the Tree of Knowledge. There are two Great Trees in Paradise, the other one called Life.

"Eat from any of the trees except for the Tree of the Knowledge of Good and Evil, because if you eat from its fruit, you will die."

The Man smiles. "There are plenty of other trees of so many kinds! We will never hunger."

So for measureless time before time has any real meaning, the Man and Woman enjoy life in Paradise. One day while the Man takes a nap, the Woman wanders closer to the Tree of Knowledge, whose fruit the Creator forbade them to eat.

Suddenly she draws back, a bit startled, for in the shade against the trunk is leaning another two-legged creature, though unlike herself and her husband, this one gleams with a smooth cool skin that shows an elegant pattern of scales. Plus his eyes are as round as the Moon and the Sun. "Let us walk in the Garden and talk," it says.

"Who are you?" she says.

"I am called the Serpent."

"Why have I never seen you before?"

"Well, I am quite good at remaining concealed, at only being seen when I wish to be seen."

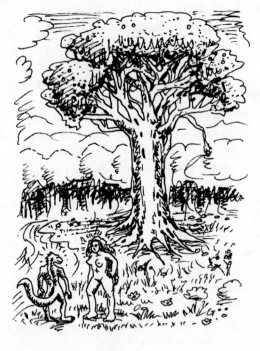

The Serpent and the Woman in the Garden

"This is the Tree of the Knowledge of Good and Evil, the One Tree that the Creator told us we must not eat the fruit of... or we will die!"

The Serpent steps forward into the light. "Do you believe that?" His body shimmers and shines, it ripples with his muscular grace, though a forked tongue quite unlike that of the Man, her husband, flickers forth from his snout, and then withdraws again.

"Believe... ? How can I imagine that anything the Creator told us was not true?"

"You will not die if you eat the fruit on the branches above me here. Oh no, not at all! Rather, your eyes will be opened and you will see everything as it really is for the first time. You will live forever and be more like the Creator. You will see that in reality you are also gods!"

"How can I believe you? This could not be worth the risk of death!"

"What I tell you is the truth, Woman. You will not die, if you eat this. You will be more like the Creator, for this is something that he withholds from you."

"Yes, I suppose it would be quite wonderful to be more like the Creator! He comes and goes from this place as he wishes. He made everything."

"Go ahead and try it. Then, when you realize that it cannot harm you, offer some to your husband. He will thank you forever after that, for your suggestion."

"Only," she hesitates, "will this not be disobedience to the Creator?"

"Follow your own heart, dear Woman."

The standard outcome of this encounter is familiar to a great many people, particularly in the Western World. And yet, though the Serpent was "punished" by the Creator, being forced to crawl along the ground limbless thereafter, and to be feared by humans, in reality serpents are not evil. Nor do they suffer due to their designated mode of moving, which works exceedingly well for them.

Indeed, in these oldest versions of the Garden Story, the Serpent is wise and subtle. It actually serves as an evolutionary messenger. As such, the "expulsion" from Paradise need not be viewed as punishment or disaster. Rather it can be recognized as a necessary emergence of humanity from our ancestors' natural state of participation mystique, undistinguished from our surroundings and from what happened to us.

Their original awareness of connection with everything in the natural world has not survived intact into the highly civilized, human-created environments of modern urban landscapes. Yet the emergence from the Garden also led to the enrichment of our minds, as we began a radical learning curve, and the astounding legacy of our inventiveness and our arts is not entirely about the warfare and destruction of recent times.

There is also a great deal of artfulness, craft, ingenuity, skill, creativity, persistence, concern for the well-being of others, community, culture, literature, science, the fine arts, and many technological advances that benefit all of humanity and the planet.

The disengagement of the mind from its Source in Nature, serves a purpose of self-awareness, yet only to the point where the self chooses deliberately to return into a harmonious reconciliation with its origins in the greater Self of Nature.

The phallic significance for you: Reclaim your Original Innocence! The doctrine of Original Sin has no basis in reality, and it derives from much later patriarchal revisions of the Garden Story designed to blame females for the weaknesses of males, to control people by controlling their natural sexual nature, and to impose generational guilt and shame.

The concept of Original Sin, the belief that you were born flawed and with inherent evil due to the sins of your ancestors, is simply untrue. In reality, you were born in the state of Original Innocence, as a sort of *tabula rasa* or a blank slate, despite the fact that much of your individuality has a genetic basis. The truth is that when you are willing to accept 100% responsibility for everything that shows up in your reality, as the co-creator of it because you participate in its creation, you gain genuine freedom!

Your pure natural sexuality in the state of Original Innocence remains intact within the layers of personal history and cultural conditioning that may confuse the issue. The most effective way to regain your Original Innocence is not through traditional psychological therapies or counseling. More effective is to learn to generate sustained and prolonged states of high quality erotic ecstasy that will dissolve those acquired blocks to happiness.

In truth, the Tree of Knowledge is that dualistic view that judges and leads to such extreme beliefs as good and evil, and even to the idea of two trees in the Garden. The truth is there is only One Tree.

Your own phallus IS the Tree of Life, the One Tree, as you will know for certain once you fully grasp the Secret of the Golden Phallus.

Male Mysteries of the Desert Dwellers

As mentioned above, the Semitic tribes native to those regions took refuge in Egypt to the west several times during periods of drought and famine in the Middle East. They returned to their homelands with some of the influences of Egyptian civilization. They also continued to encounter those who traded with India, as well as other civilized city-dwellers.

Early on, some of the men who became patriarchal leaders still practiced rituals that their descendents would come to consider sacrilegious. An example is the tradition of consulting Oracular Trees, such as the Terebinth Tree of Moreh in the land of Canaan, where sacrifices were made, as the petitioners sought omens from the gods.

There was another important grove of sacred Terebinth Trees at Mamre. This was not actual worship of the trees, rather it reflects a kind of pantheistic or animistic reverence for the spirits of the trees. And trees, being mighty vertical beings are always phallic in nature, even when the tree is biologically female as in some cases.

Though those male leaders, or patriarchs, viewed themselves as being in charge, and demanded obedience from all lower ranking men, women and children, in reality their women in particular showed tremendous strength. Often the women's quiet resolve and patient endurance proved far more effective to deal with serious problems than the competitive, possessive and warlike temperaments of the men of their tribes.

During these periods, people of the region embraced a variety of beliefs: some venerated many gods; some still held a Great Mother Goddess supreme; others now spoke of a single, invisible Lord Almighty with a tendency to help his people but also to test their faith and obedience severely at times. This monotheistic deity was probably partly inspired by Aten of Egypt, however he was given sterner, warrior-like qualities as well by those people more inclined to fear and appease their gods than the happy, celebratory Egyptians.

One of the early patriarchs was visited by three men who turned out to be messengers of the Lord Almighty, on their way to dish out punishment to a city of evildoers. Those three can be recognized archetypally as an incarnation of the Triple God, who is so important in the Male Mysteries.

Another time the same patriarch was instructed to sacrifice his own first-born son. However at the last moment as he had raised the knife, the account tells that a messenger of the Lord Almighty told him not to do it, and pointed out a sacrificial animal nearby.

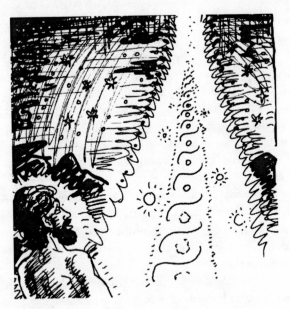

A Vision of the Stairway to Heaven

Another great patriarch dreamed of seeing a "Ladder to the Sky" with heavenly messengers passing up and down—definitely a vision of the World Axis that connects Below with Above, a cosmic phallus. The same patriarch, on at least five occasions pushed upright large stones, in honor of his God, then anointed the stones with oil. This clearly echoes the East Indian rites of venerating Shiva-lingam by pouring oblations over an upright stone phallus.

Certain miraculous events and granted boons did indeed seem to accompany obedience and faith in this invisible and often stern God. Sometimes patriarchs lived immensely long lives, and their wives might prove to be fertile and bear young long after they thought they were past a childbearing age. Though monotheistic, these tribes were not monogamous, and the matter of men consorting with lesser wives and concubines to provide offspring on behalf of barren wives often became an issue of contention.

In relation to Egypt, some of the most fabulous accounts arose...

A great leader of the tribe encounters the Lord Almighty while he tends a flock of sheep in the desert. He observes a shrub that appears to be burning, yet is not consumed, instead, it radiates heat and light.

A voice says, "Take off your shoes...you are standing on holy ground."

"Who or what are you?" the man asks.

The answer comes: "I AM what I AM becoming."

Then this unseen Lord Almighty demands that the man act on his behalf, and the man tries to get out of it. Instead, he is given a miraculous sign to perform so that he might be believed when he speaks of this experience.

"Throw down your staff."

When he does so, the staff became a serpent.

"Now, pick it up by the tail," the voice instructs.

Though he feels terrified, the man obeys, and the serpent becomes his staff again.

The sign of empowerment this man received can be understood for what it means in its essence: the staff represents his spine, and the serpent is the yogic Serpent Power, the life force. The same basic image, a staff entwined by the Serpent Power, would later become the caduceus, the staff of Hermes, the Greek Messenger of the Gods. Likewise as the thyrsus of Dionysus, celebrants recreated the image with a pinecone mounted on a staff entwined with green ivy. Again, this is the universal axis: the power of the phallus, which is the same as the World Tree archetype, that connects Below with Above.

The World Tree is also the vegetative higher intelligence within the matrix of the biosphere that we sometimes call Gaia. According to science, the blue-green algae, the plant kingdom and the fungi are elders and ancestors of multi-celled animals such as humans. In fact, the DNA wisdom of the vegetative intelligence feeds all living things on Earth, maintains the balance of gases in the atmosphere, and circulates the moisture and the air upon which all living things depend.

All of these images are essentially the same phallic realities: the World Tree or Tree of Life; the staff entwined with a serpent; the human spine, upright and activated by the Serpent Power of erotic energy; the axis of the world, the vertical energy that connects Below with Above, Earth with Sky; the Cosmic Phallus of the Triple God.

Clearly the shrub blazing yet unconsumed IS the Tree of Life. In fact, there has always been only this One Tree in archetypal essence. All actual trees are incarnations of this essential One Tree of Life. It is likewise your own Sacred Phallus. To realize this is to return to living in the Paradise Garden, and to recover your Original Innocence.

Later when this same patriarch who spoke with the vegetative higher intelligence through the radiant, unconsumed shrub led his people from Egypt to a new home in the Middle East, he was guided by the vision of "a pillar of cloud by day, and a pillar of fire by night." These images clearly represent the familiar World Axis, the same energetic reality that his own forefather saw as a luminous pathway that connected Earth with Sky.

Something that makes those men of ancient times quite admirable in some ways is their willingness to listen to what they consider the voice and signs of their Lord Almighty. Unfortunately, it seems they could not always distinguish that voice from their own unconscious agendas, which were sometimes vengeful and judgmental.

Here we also see the advent of the unfortunate belief that this monotheistic deity will punish bad behavior or reward good behavior. Such moralistic judgment and partiality reflects the parental quality of a deity that treats people like children that require strict guidance. This departs from the kind of personal empowerment in which you are encouraged to make your own choices based upon inner integrity.

In today's world, psychological studies reveal overwhelmingly that punishment is not an effective means to improve a person's behavior. Encouragement, praise, and fostering good self-esteem and self-image, and self-reward however, are effective to help a person achieve greater balance and lasting happiness.

It may seem trite, still this is true: to love yourself is the key to loving others in a balanced, harmonious manner. Thus when any tradition, and this includes almost all major cultures and religions of today's world, tries to manipulate behaviors through shame and guilt, they become coercive rather than empowering. They advocate power over others, rather than power from within. They actually make things worse.

In today's world we live on a planet fundamentally different from the one around 4000 years ago, or about 2000 BCE, described in the accounts of the monotheistic patriarchs above.

Today our planet evolves rapidly toward a radical shift. The rate of change of every kind accelerates exponentially. This includes technological advance, computing speed, population growth, and environmental challenges.

Mathematicians call this immanent shift the Singularity. We cannot precisely anticipate the near future, any more than weather forecasters know for sure what the weather will be like tomorrow.

The Singularity is a shift so radical we cannot anticipate its nature, and yet we might as well imagine it to be a good shift of consciousness, and evolutionary quantum leap towards planetary awareness and reconciliation with Nature itself. To imagine it this way may, instead of with fears of doomsday, will help the change to manifest in the direction of a better future for the species and our world.

The math is compelling. In the year 1804 the Earth's human population reached one billion for the first time; by 1930 it doubled to two billion people; in the 1960s, it was around three billion; now we number about seven billion; by 2050, who knows?

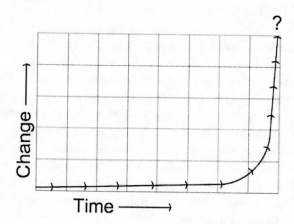

Approaching Singularity

See how the rate of change curves up the other arm of the graph?

When it nearly parallels that arm, we approach Singularity.

The phallic significance for you: Rather than fear of the future, let these realities inspire wonder and awe, as we face both the greatest challenges our species has ever created, and the greatest opportunities. By becoming a phallic god, you do your part for humanity and the planet.

Rather than confront the drawbacks of patriarchal and monotheistic cultures, your own growth is more effectively served by a simple shift to the loving embrace of the Male Mysteries and Phallic Brotherhood. Undertake a course of devoted study of Male Erotic Alchemy and allow it to transform you. Learn and practice the ways to generate the finest erotic ecstasy until it becomes Golden Phallus Yoga.

Rather than question those ancient heritages, simply turn your attention to listen deeply to the innate wisdom that comes now and here from your own penis. Sufficient ecstasy will gradually evaporate all acquired guilt and shame over nakedness, sexuality and your penis. Nothing is more sacred that your body and your enjoyment of it.

Our species is not good or bad: *WE ARE what WE ARE becoming.*

I AM: The Divine IS in Your Hands

Most traditions that persist for more than a few years become control structures designed to preserve and protect their own continuation. In this manner, the first known bureaucracies can be traced to 18th Dynasty Egypt, when for the first time a standing military existed in the Two Lands.

The horse, the chariot and the long-bow had recently been imported into Egypt from the Middle East, along with some families of foreign warriors who could train Egyptians in the uses of these new military technologies. So a new treasury to administer the military was created. Though the Egyptians had no form of money such as a symbolic currency, for many centuries the people had been taxed in the form of certain percentages of goods that were collected by the temple treasuries.

The temple treasuries had controlled all the wealth of the Two Lands for the first millennia or more of the culture's existence. The ancient kings, rulers later called pharaoh, or "Great House," in practice owned the Two Lands as the Good God, the Living Image of Osiris, who was called the Great God. Usually without question, the temples provided the divine rulers with whatever they wanted.

However a new division arose during the 18th Dynasty. A new set of scribes was created to administer the tributes collected and designated for the military, when before these "taxes" had only been for the pharaoh and for the temples.

Texts of correspondence between Egyptian rulers and foreign rulers reveal the division of interests that arose. In classic form the bureaucrat swiftly took on the primary job of perpetuating his own office and the institution of the bureaucracy, rather than the stated purpose of the bureau. That purpose became secondary, as it still is today.

Men designated as scribes became ruthless enforcers of official policy, a guise for operatives that has changed little in over three millennia since then.

Seemingly any human organization of more than twelve or thirteen people tends to automatically become hierarchical, as it grows unwieldy to operate according to a consensus of equals. Plus, when a remarkable individual displays a special connection with the Source of All Things, and manifests unusual wisdom that comes directly from that connection, people usually find such an individual highly attractive, or quite threatening. The people attracted to such an individual likewise almost always fail to really grasp what that individual actually experiences and seeks to convey.

The followers interpret the experience through their own filters, and through their own familiar paradigm. In this manner, those who recorded the teachings of Lord Buddha had come out of an ancient Vedic and Hindu paradigm. They inevitably interpreted his teachings as was possible for them. Jesus taught his radical path of love and forgiveness among Hebrews of a Greek-flavored world under Roman domination.

Understandably, the original messages rapidly grew obscured and even got lost in the dramatic historical shuffle of the following centuries. Eventually wars were fought in the name of Christ, which Jesus would not have appreciated at all with his teachings of radical love, forgiveness and non-violence.

Lord Buddha offered clear psychological insights into the cause of suffering. He denied the existence of a supernatural and insisted all experience had a mental basis. Yet to his teachings were added far older concepts of reincarnation and karma from precious lifetimes, whose supernatural nature the Buddha would not have accepted.

To the powerful wisdom that life can be transformed by choosing not to return negativity to those who might treat you badly, the early Christian church added all kinds of beliefs concerning the afterlife of reward and punishment, sexual taboos, and dualistic concepts of good and evil, all of which long predated Jesus and were not part of his actual message of awakening to Love.

Though more skeptical scholars consider the gospel narratives up to the baptism with serious doubt, the flight to Egypt and return from there to Nazareth seems plausible, given how Jesus seemed to deliberately live out the passion of Osiris.

In fact, the original Holy Family or Trinity of Egypt was Isis and Osiris and their son Horus. Clearly the life of Jesus echoed the core Mysteries of the Egyptian religion that centered on Osiris, Isis and their Holy Child. Similar life stories and similar names are related to a continuity of teachers who lived out the "dying god" archetype and were said to have returned to life.

Tammuz, Dumuzi, Osiris, Horus, Adonis, Dionysus, Jesus…

Major organized religions inevitably lose their way as they stray far from the intentions of the figures they are founded around. Still, a clear-eyed, open-minded examination with an open heart reveals some spiritual treasures from all traditions.

Great human beings can inspire you when you obtain a glimpse of the mystery of human existence and unknown potentials. It seems anything may be possible! Life becomes a grand adventure of discovery, just as small children often view everyday life.

All of the mysteries are alive within you. Divine nature is not only in you, but also in everyone and everything else. It cannot be located somewhere more than anywhere else, nor is it subject to description, understanding, or personification.

A courageous, clear view accepts the challenge to recognize the Divine in everyone and everything. To acknowledge that everything is alive; everything is sacred! Once you begin to consider all things as sacred, you not only inhabit a living planet, you are part of a living universe. Everything circles back to a sensible, awesome spirituality of wonder and gratitude for the sheer fact of your own existence!

Oneness that includes all concepts of divinity.
Nothing rewards or punishes you but you.
You live in a supportive Universe.
You are the I AM.

Was Jesus a Male Erotic Alchemist?

There is much we may never know for sure about the historical man now known as Jesus of Nazareth. Yet a careful reading of the *New Testament* and examination of other evidence such as the controversial *Secret Gospel of Mark* suggests that Jesus may have employed a process similar to Male Erotic Alchemy to initiate some of his followers.

To consider this case, we need not assume that he was what we now call a "gay" man, with a primary same-sex attraction. However, the circumstantial evidence, based on the likelihood that at least some narrative elements of the gospels are accurate, does suggest this possibility.

Evidently Jesus spent most of his public career surrounded by an intimate group of male disciples, the entourage tended and cared for by a small group of devoted women who traveled with them. Also, the qualities of deep understanding of human nature from the "outsider's perspective," along with profound empathy, a marked distaste for conflict, and brilliant skills as an entertaining storyteller and communicator, a profoundly loving man who loved everyone and the world itself, are all quite commonly characteristics of men we now call "gay."

Certain non-canonical fragments of text are also highly suggestive. The *Gospel According to Thomas* was discovered at Nag Hammadi, Egypt in 1945. This collection of 114 sayings attributed to Jesus is perhaps the earliest fragment of gospel in existence, for it was actually written down in the 1st Century CE, within living memory of Jesus. There is no narrative to speak of, rather it records dialogue between Jesus, his followers and sometimes his audience.

Thomas reveals a quite different and probably far more accurate glimpse of the actual man's teachings than those recorded in the much later canonical texts. There is no mention of crucifixion, resurrection, final judgment, or any messianic notions about Jesus; rather he is presented as a great and revolutionary teacher. His message in *Thomas* is one of love and forgiveness, and that *this* world can be experienced as the Kingdom of Heaven for those "with eyes to see and ears to hear."

Many open-minded scholars now do consider this text to be valuable corrective feedback on the more distorted and later *New Testament* accounts. Far more controversial however, is a brief fragment known as *The Secret Gospel of Mark*. In 2004, scholar Will Roscoe published *Jesus and the Shamanic Tradition of Same-Sex Love,* a meticulous and revolutionary examination of this text and its implications.

Secret Mark as a whole may have originally been an earlier and more complete version of what is now known as *The Gospel of Mark*. The only direct quote from *Secret Mark* cited in Roscoe's book is a brief passage quoted in what appears to be a letter from Clement of Alexandria (circa. 150-215 CE). In the letter, Clement denounces the practices of a group of early Christians who apparently performed certain homoerotic rites mentioned in *Secret Mark*. Roscoe carefully unravels the evidence that indicates Jesus may have employed a private erotic initiation with men to provide them with a taste of the Kingdom of Heaven on Earth.

Clearly this initiation is not only sexual, but about Love, in the sense of Phallic Brotherhood. It also does not indicate that this was the primary teaching of Jesus, rather that it may have been among the methods he employed to give some followers an experience of divine bliss. As radical as this may seem in today's context, in the ancient world of two millennia past and among tribal and hunter-gatherer peoples, such an initiatory rite would not seem so controversial or unusual.

For all we truly know, Jesus may also have been married and had children, as some other current interpretations propose. Through most of history, and in various parts of the world even now, many married men sincerely love their wives and children, while for purely erotic enjoyment, they may consort with fellow males. Often this is rationalized as not even being unfaithful or adulterous, as the husband is not having sex with another woman! In fact, by now there may be many thousands of living descendants of Jesus on Planet Earth.

Aside from the later additions to the *New Testament* of certain teachings that seem misogynistic and homophobic, even in the canonical gospel accounts, Jesus himself never speaks of sexuality at all, except to say that adultery is a bad idea, and that if you sin lustfully in your thoughts, you actually sin. Apart from the anti-sexual bias of some later interpreters, the actual teachings focus on responsible and loving treatment of others, not specific sexual activities.

Given what we now understand about the cultivation of male erotic energy as a means of personal growth and conscious evolution, we can speculate that Jesus may have been a Male Erotic Alchemist and that he sometimes spent a night alone with another man to share high erotic states for their mutual benefit and uplifting.

Your Penis IS the One Tree

Your human design is said to be created in the image of the Creator. What does this truly mean?

Stories in themselves are just mind-stuff, mental imagery that you may find entertaining. You might even learn something from them—however stories only really come alive and have powerful significance when you totally absorb and digest them, when they become part of you. When you know that they are essentially about you.

When you digest a story like delicious, nourishing food and it becomes part of you, a story is no longer merely a mind-game, rather it speaks to your cells and from your cells simultaneously.

All the stories in this book offer important awareness of what it is to be embodied as a human male on the planet at this time. The stories and images tell you things beyond the words themselves about those ancestors within you. You are empowered to accept the glorious and mysterious gift of your embodiment and your penis with the sense of wonder and awe that is their due.

In essence, the Secret of the Golden Phallus is extremely simple. To experience this reality is not complicated. However, it does require the humility of admitting to yourself that you may have missed the point of having a penis and being a human male in a body—until now! Now all the gaps begin to fill in, the dots connect.

This requires only surrender, and the willingness to start over again each and every time you gaze along your torso to the base of your belly, to regard that miraculous, highly-evolved male organ rooted between your legs, and every time, you lovingly manipulate your penis with those amazing opposable-thumbed and highly dexterous human hands.

The final piece to this process of fully digesting the phallic stories about forefathers and ancestors, humans and gods and demons and monsters, is to accept your own divine nature.

Your body reflects the universal design and is magnificently designed. Along the middle axis that parallels your spine from the sacrum to the crown of your skull, your torso and limbs overall have a bilateral form. This means the left and right halves reflect each other. Internally this holds true a great deal in your legs and arms, particularly in terms of skeletal structure, muscles, tendons and ligaments, and the intricate weavings of the circulatory and nervous systems.

Your central nervous system is comprised of your spinal column and brain. In itself this has a tree-like form, a lengthy trunk rises from the tapered root, then branches where it meets the brain at the brain stem, into a neurological "canopy" or treetop of immense complexity. This overall form also resembles a mushroom, those fruiting bodies of the mycelium so crucial to the rich and living soils of forested regions. The microorganisms and threadlike fibers of the mycelial weave in the soil resemble your peripheral nervous system elaborated beyond your brain and spine through the rest of your body. Your embodied nature perfectly reflects Nature itself.

Return your attention to those aspects of your design that are singular and that closely follow the central axis of your body from root to crown: your anus, your penis, your navel, generally your heart, and precisely your head. All else extends in reflective symmetry left and right from this central axis.

Your penis reflects both a tree and all of Nature in its structure.
Your penile shaft is the trunk, the glans is the canopy.
It is also the World Tree, the *Axis mundi*.
There is only One Tree: Life.
Feel it.

CHAPTER FIVE:

THE MALE MYSTERIES OF EUROPE

A common assumption is that Europe and the Western World owes much of its historical and cultural basis to ancient Greece. Indeed the Greek philosophers laid much of the groundwork for modern science and art, plus the Athenian experiment inspired our modern concept of democratic government.

However, we owe many even deeper and more widespread innovations to the ancient Egyptians, the first people to sit on chairs at tables, to write on paper, and to commonly live with those felines we call "domestic" cats, which actually domesticated people and themselves remain somewhat wild animals.

Plus the Egyptians created the first truly phallocentric culture.

The great civilization of Egypt had long ago passed its peak and was already waning when the brilliance of the Greeks arose across the Mediterranean Sea to the north. From around 700 to 300 BCE those great city-states of Athens and Sparta flourished, as well as outposts of the same basic culture on many nearby islands and along the coast of Asia Minor to the East.

From Macedonia just north of the Greek heartland, arose the Great Alexander, who conquered much of the known world—including part of India—during his brief lifetime, inspired by his famous teacher Aristotle. The myth of Shiva's first son, Skanda, the patron of homosexual men, became connected with Alexander, and their names are related.

Alexander's teacher Aristotle was the last and third of a remarkable legacy of great philosophers that began with Socrates and his student Plato.

Philosophy means literally "the love of wisdom," and those early philosophers sought to understand the nature of the world and the place of humans in the scheme of things. Though they lacked our technological tools, they laid the groundwork for scientific enquiry, which continues to flourish and produces extraordinary information, theories, and technological innovations.

As significant and pervasive as science in today's world, however, is the mythic and religious heritage of the Greeks, whose ancient stories of Creation, and of the gods and goddesses forms a visual, symbolic and linguistic vocabulary that pervades Western culture and has also spread to the East.

Many major philosophers, such as the mathematician and mystic Pythagoras, were influenced by ancient Egyptian teachings, and some actually traveled to Egypt and studied there. Likewise, many of the Greek myths and symbols and gods have roots in ancient Egypt. The early Greeks themselves enjoyed a strong phallocentric tendency. They honored the phallus and celebrated phallic festivals.

Less admirably the Greeks became so male dominant that women suffered far lower status than in Egypt, where women remained honored and equal to men.

At every crossroads in ancient Greece, and at the major entrances of public buildings, stood a shrine called a "Herm." This honored Hermes, the messenger of the gods. The Herm usually took the form of a vertical pillar topped by the bearded head of a man and from the surface of the pillar below the head, an erect phallus protruded.

The Herm probably originated from the Egyptian phallic image of Lord Menu, the Valley God, depicted as a standing, bearded king with simplified body, one arm raised, the other hand holding his erect phallus. Lord Menu's figure may have been simplified further to become the simple pillar of the Herm.

Hermes was the patron of young men, associated with gymnasiums where Greek males sported naked, where older men watched athletes in action. Hermes had various roles, for he also served as a guide for souls of the deceased to the Underworld, he sponsored commerce, protected thieves, was god of crossroads and also all border crossings.

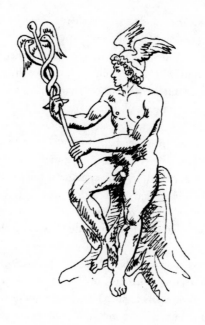

Hermes of the Crossroads

Crossroads and borders are where the living and the dead meet.
Menu was the phallic god of regeneration, patron of Osiris.
Osiris was Lord of the Dead and King of Eternity.
Osiris resurrected himself via masturbation.
Read between the lines and absorb.
Look between your legs.
Smile!

Greek Phallicism and Male Dominance

During the last millennium or two BCE most of the goddess-oriented imagery and stories was overturned or at least revised in favor of patriarchal gods, and in the later stages these became the stern, often warlike monotheistic Gods of male dominance.

This may have started somewhat innocently, when men became envious of the powerful Female Mysteries of the women. In goddess-oriented cultures, the women sometimes actually experienced their menstrual cycles not only in synchrony with other women, but also synchronized with the natural lunar cycle of thirteen Moons or "months," in a remarkable linkage of human experience with natural process.

This, of course is why menstruation is sometimes termed a woman's "monthlies." This wonderful—perhaps to many men uncanny—link with Nature perpetuated the sisterly solidarity of women in those situations where matricentrist values persisted. In such situations, the partnership choices of women, motherhood itself, and child rearing were protected and considered sacrosanct. There is no evidence of women dominating, as in the myths of the Amazons, however in matricentrist cultures female values were honored and protected.

This began to change with the spread of both warrior technologies such as the riding of horses, wheeled chariots, more advanced weapons like the longbow, and agriculture, all of which led to the founding of cities and urban cultures anchored in husbandry, agriculture, and organized warfare.

Though the somewhat migratory lifestyles of many hunter-gatherer tribes persisted, and a few of them even survive today, the urbanized, male-dominant, militarized modes of human civilization succeeded and thrived, for better or for worse, and mostly for worse.

Male dominance unleashed much suffering and destruction. Aggressive tendencies were institutionalized as the cults of warrior gods. Male ownership of women and children in the guise of marriage, and also homophobia became widely sanctioned as "natural." Agriculture led to overpopulation and changed people's relationship with the landscape leading to ownership and conflict.

The dark side of agriculture is that it has also led to poor nutrition with an over-emphasis on refined carbohydrate products and sugar, and now the environmental devastation from petrochemical pesticides and fertilizers, as well as GMOs.

Though oppressive patriarchal and monotheistic beliefs emerged that continue to limit the lives of billions of people today—it was not all bad. Far from it. Like all radical innovations, tremendous advances also resulted. The consequences were mixed.

In practice, women have remained covertly somewhat in control though mostly from behind the scenes. Otherwise the aggressive male-dominators would probably have already killed everybody and destroyed everything. Women, who have strong instincts for motherhood and sisterhood hard-wired, are those who put on the brakes when men get totally out of control. Then, women say, "No! This is my son, my brother, my father. You will not torture or kill him. It's time to stop this violent game and take a break."

At this turning point in the planet's life, it's important that women assume more leadership roles, not in domination of men, but in full and balanced partnership.

No such ideal partnership existed in ancient Greece.

In that period the women maintained strong influence over their men, as the myths and dramas, both tragedies and comedies reveal. However women in Greece were mostly kept hidden in the household, to serve as wives and mothers, with the only real alternative for women being prostitution.

Still, the Greeks did honor and celebrate the phallus in ways that were not always oppressive to women. Phallic charms, talismans and amulets proliferated to ward of the "evil eye," or curses. The erect penis was powerful good juju! Greek festivals sometimes involved carrying around huge wood and leather phallic images in procession, making music, and drumming and dancing around with a lot of orgiastic carrying on.

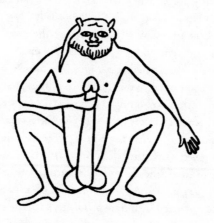

A Satyr Masturbating in the Woodlands

During the rites of Dionysus, wine was used as a potent drug to release inhibitions. Women chased men and whacked them with the thyrsus to enact the frenzy of the Maenads who tore apart the god Dionysus by chasing men and whacking them with the thyrsus. *Ouch!* A pinecone on a stick can be painful!

Also the satyrs—mythically half-goat wild men associated with the Great God Pan and the nymphs—were actual men who haunted the woodlands, often naked and engaged in orgiastic rites, to honor the fertility of Nature Spirits. Such practices were not merely symbolic for the Greeks, they were actual and served to help maintain a real connection with Nature as the culture grew increasingly urbanized. The famous images painted on pottery of masturbating satyrs preserves an actual experiential part of the culture that allowed for such natural and healthy behavior, at least in certain contexts.

However the unusual tolerance for homosexual behavior in ancient Greece was not actually a modern gay man's fantasy free-for-all. For the most part, male relationships between adult men of similar ages were frowned upon. Sparta's famed army of pairs of male lovers was a notable exception to this.

The institution of formalized male love in Greece was formulaic: an older married man could properly act as a mentor and sponsor to a teenage youth. The older man formally assumed responsibility for the education and proper development of the young man in all ways, physically, intellectually, and spiritually. The younger man often, if not always, was expected to express his gratitude with erotic favors for his older, usually bearded mentor. After the young man began to show a beard, which the Greeks called "clouds covering the Sun," the relationship was expected to end.

The youth would enter manhood, grow his own beard and marry; in turn he became a sponsor of younger men. The onset of a young man's first beard they called, "Clouds covering the Sun." **This formula of youth and age in cycles for male relationships was not for a small subset of men considered homosexual, *rather most men practiced something like this!* It confirms that given social sanction, the majority of men can naturally appreciate some kind of erotic connection with fellow males. The current estimates of 10% gay men and a larger portion of bisexual men is clearly conservative and distorted by innate problems with the research methods of polling and interviews. Obviously male sexuality is a spectrum without clearcut divisions!** In ancient Greece, a large proportion of the men engaged in same-sex relations, as well as usually being married, as those were the social paradigms.

Though the Greek institution was not exactly today's concept of homosexual love, the Greeks did enjoy healthy attitudes with the institution of the gymnasium. In this context, young men, athletes, and warriors exercised and practiced their martial arts in the nude, and usually before an appreciative audience of older men.

Hermes patronized this kind of fraternal nudity and the healthy male bonding involved.

The Secret Origins of Pan

According to the later patriarchal versions of the Greek myths, Hermes was the father of the woodland god Pan, the goat-legged phallic god said to live in the woodlands of Arcadia on the Peloponnesus Peninsula. Yet this does not really make sense, as Pan is clearly a primordial deity allied with the oldest and deepest instinctual forces of Nature. Hermes, dazzling and handsome as he may be, is one of those lofty, much later Olympians. Of course, Zeus tried to claim responsibility for everything important, and Pan remained popular into more recent times.

The first clue to the truth is the matter of Hermes's job as messenger god, a job taken from the goddess Iris, and given to him instead. She was of an earlier generation of the elder gods. She served Hera, the wife of Zeus. As such, Iris, the Rainbow Goddess, connected Earth and Sky, and traveled fast as the wind, even into the depth of the sea and the Underworld.

The winged staff entwined with two serpents, called the caduceus, that Hermes later carried, originally belonged to Iris. Her husband was Zephyrus, god of the West Wind. Iris personified the rainbow itself, and represented the full spectrum of possibilities that connects everything from the lowest to the highest.

There is no clear account of why Zeus gave her job to his son Hermes, except that it seems part of the patriarchal conversion that sought to diminish the importance of all goddesses. Zeus philandered frequently, seldom able to avoid the notice of his jealous wife, Hera, the Queen of Heaven. During one such tryst, with Maia, a nymph sometimes call the Goddess of Spring, the

Lord of Sky engendered his son Hermes. Because Hermes was one of her husband's bastards, Hera never appreciated Hermes.

Later stories reassigned other maternities to Hermes, and said that he himself engendered Lord Pan with Maia.

In reality, Hermes did not marry, being of an athletic and male-companion-oriented nature. Regardless of this, once given the caduceus of Iris along with her job, Hermes did indeed travel faster and farther than any of his somewhat reclusive family who all spent a great deal of their time ensconced within the fabulous Palace of Zeus Thunderer atop Mount Olympus.

Pan of Arcadia, however, the Woodland God who is Lord of Forest and Field, was a far more ancient and primordial deity than any of the Olympians. The oldest version of his parentage ultimately returns to the previous generations of divinities before the Olympians, the Titans or the Elder Gods, and Gaia's Beloved Monsters…

Lord Kronus, King of the Titans, has driven his father Uranus back into the Sky. Remember: Gaia helps Kronus to accomplish this, after his promise to release her Beloved Monsters from the Underworld, and then he assumes power as Lord of Sky.

Like his father, unfortunately Kronus not only forgets that promise, he similarly wanders far and wide to copulate with almost anyone or anything he can find to do it with. He discovers the monstrous she-goat called Aix, one of Gaia's Beloved Monsters, who had avoided banishment by living in the remote wilds of Arcadia. Kronus mounts Aix as well, though once he climaxes, he immediately flees from their cataclysmic mating.

Aix is left to give birth to the half-goat godling Pan. Like any godling, Pan matures swiftly to become the full-grown satyr form familiar to most of the world, even today. However Pan remains totally a wild thing, for once he is weaned, his monstrous mother drives him away to find his own part of the woodlands to live in.

Pan almost always sports a huge erection, and through all of his early existence he desperately seeks partners with whom to couple, such as nymphs, shepherdesses and shepherds, even goats and other animals. In this, he resembles his father Kronus. Anything in the least bit willing, Pan engages in erotic sport with. Many are the stories of demi-gods and mortals terrified into flight when alone in the woodlands…

Hermes eventually discovers Pan in the woodlands of Arcadia, playing plaintively upon the syrinx, a pipe of reeds he fashioned himself from rushes that grew along a shoreline where the nymph Syrinx, in flight from him had cried out for help, and was transformed by Hera into a bed of reeds.

By this time Pan has been living for a very long time in the woodlands. His only companion most of the time is a drunken old satyr called Silenus.

As yet, the current Queen of Heaven, Hera, knows nothing about the Woodland God until her stepson Hermes brings him up to the marble halls of Olympus to visit. "Who is this noisy and odorous creature?" Hera says, eyes wide and nose turned up.

Indeed, Pan's hooves clatter on the hard marble floors as he walks and he smells strongly, though it is a sweet natural fragrance, and some golden bees buzz around him.

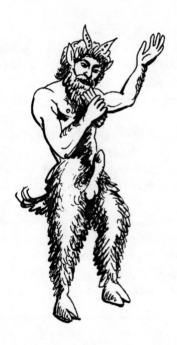

Pan in Arcadia

"His name is Pan," Hermes says, "and he lives in the woodlands of Arcadia."

"I don't recognize this fellow, however he is rather amusing," Hera says, and with the rest of her family, the other gods and goddesses of Olympus, she laughs.

The Olympians do not mean to be cruel, however they often feel high above and beyond concerns over the feelings and everyday experience of all that lives below their lofty home.

Hermes realizes that he made a mistake to bring Pan up there, and immediately returns him to his home, a place that Hermes actually finds more delightful and fun than his father's mountaintop mansion.

"I'm sorry if my family and their household laughed at you," Hermes says.

Pan shrugs and grins. "Laughter is a good thing, my handsome young friend! You have shown me a place where I would not want to live, even if I was invited to dwell there with my own staff of servants to do my bidding."

Hermes looks upon him with admiration shining in his face, his fists planted on his narrow hips, the caduceus in one hand. His splendid youthful nakedness shines upon the forest greenery and trees.

"You are a most sensible and admirable fellow," Hermes says. "I will not forget you, and I hope that you will be my friend from now on."

"But of course," Pan tells him.

The phallic significance for you: Your own phallic nature is an ancient part of your animal heritage, a great gift, and something to be honored in the right context. Human civilizations long ago sometimes held a place for the Male Mysteries, however much has changed in the last few thousand years. Despite many good advances, serious problems have arisen from people's alienation from Nature itself and from the natural eroticism of our biological heritage.

Now it is crucial to regain your authentic, shameless, guilt-free erotic nature. There may always be contexts in which this is not appreciated. So seek out and spend time in environments secluded, or private enough, by yourself or in the company of sympathetic souls where your authentic phallic nature can be experienced and celebrated.

The woodlands, forests and fields are a great place to be naked and aroused.

What Hermes Taught Pan

It may seem that some things have always existed, such as the Universe and masturbation itself, yet in both cases, some stories tell otherwise. The story of science says that the vast complexity of this Universe burst forth from a single dimensionless point smaller than the period at the end of this sentence, about 13.7 billion years before now.

Likewise, though it maybe tough to imagine that it did not exist before then, one myth indicates that Hermes invented masturbation...

One day while awaiting the next message he is to convey on behalf of his father, the Lord of Sky, Hermes idly plays with his staff called the caduceus. For some reason, his penis begins to swell, perhaps by some kind of association. A sort of bell goes off in his head. He gazes down at his growing erection and sets the caduceus aside.

He brings both hands together between his legs...

Eventually Hermes flies down to the woodlands of Arcadia to tell his special friend the Great God Pan about his wonderful invention. His research and development phase kept reminding him of his friend, the woodland god of Arcadia, who always seems to sport a huge erection from the juncture of his shaggy legs, and who always seems to need something to do with that magnificent, raw-looking, upright thing!

Pan lives within the hollow trunk of a huge oak tree that was long ago struck by lightning, when a chamber burned out from its heart. Then it continued to grow for centuries more and formed a perfect woodland cottage-cave for Pan to live in.

One bright morning Hermes appears in the glade before Pan's dwelling place and shouts out in his young masculine voice: "Where are you, my friend, Pan?"

After a time, Pan emerges yawning and scratching his balls. "Why are you waking me up this way, young fellow?"

"Oh, I've invented something totally fantastic that I want to share with you!"

"Just so you don't want me to go with you somewhere else... I'm quite content where I AM, as I AM."

"Trust me, Friend," Hermes says, "you will thank me for sharing this with you."

Pan appears unconvinced. "Though you seem to have a lot of thieves and smugglers and pirates among your followers, I don't believe that you have ever lied to me, young sprout. So tell me."

"Better if I just show you," his handsome Olympian friend says. "Would you please bring me some olive oil?"

With a shrug, Pan goes back inside his tree. Hermes grins and goes to sit down upon a huge stump that Silenus, Faunus and a few other forest friends of the woodland god sometimes use as a sort of table or altar. He sets aside his caduceus, and as he is already naked, he begins to caress his own body with both hands.

Pan brings a jar of olive oil and places it on the ground.

Hermes's penis grows fully erect as he gazes down upon it. His hands circle over his chest, his abdomen, his hips, down his thigh and knees, over his calves, then back up the insides of his legs to converge between his legs. He caresses his genitals delicately at first, and his expression fills with joyous intent at his delicious sensations.

Then he pauses to anoint both hands with olive oil and he continues; the lubrication renders his masturbation extremely intense, and Hermes spreads his knees even wider. His pelvis rocks, his chest heaves and he sighs and moans with the intensity of his self-induced bliss. His handsome head of curly hair falls back upon the sturdy neck, eyes half-closed and mouth gaped wide. He emits deep groans and gasps of delight.

At first, Pan appears somewhat puzzled, then understanding dawns in his golden eyes. "This is amazing to see!" Pan declares. "It's something I want to feel for myself!"

Hermes stands up. His erection, shiny and stiff, bobs in front of the middle of his body. "I'm not saying this is better than making love with a goddess, or a nymph or a woman, or even with a young man, for that matter. However it's every bit as good, and perhaps better in some ways. You can enjoy this anytime and never feel needy or rejected."

"Well," Pan says, "let me anoint my hands and try this new thing."

So he does as Hermes does and the Lord of Forest and Fields is never the same god. Within moments his eyes are wild, he grins, hoots, groans and gasps in delighted amazement! While his existence has mostly been spent desperately longing for sexual fulfillment, chasing erotic pleasure and never getting quite enough even when it does happen, now Pan changes radically as he begins instead to masturbate incessantly.

"Plus, there is no reason this should be a lonely pursuit," Hermes tells him. "Let me show you how we can share it. Come here and sit beside me on this stump." He moves his seat to one side of the mossy top of the stump and Pan sits down beside him. *Hermes removes his hands from himself and reaches his closer arm across, to gently push Pan's fingers away from his erection. He takes over the honors and begins to masturbate Pan.* "Now," Hermes instructs him, "you play with mine while I play with yours."

"I feel yours as you feel mine," Pan says.

And Hermes adds, "Sharing our pleasure is Divine!"

The phallic significance for you: Explore and diversify your practice of masturbating mindfully by going into wild places such as woodlands or wilderness. Find a place of both natural beauty and privacy, get naked and pleasure yourself. Even if this is not remote, find some place as free as possible from human modification. Take with you plenty of healthy food and water to keep fed and hydrated, along with some excellent lubrication for your erection. Allow your mental processes to cease, if possible, in the intensity of sensations. Let your boundaries dissolve into a feeling of connection with Nature.

You may wish to share the powerful experience of prolonged outdoor masturbation with a phallic brother or brothers, who also enjoy Mindful Masturbation and the sharing of it. Make an agreement with your cohorts not to engage in oral or anal activity, only masturbation and touch, just for this purpose of sharing pure-hearted, innocent phallic brotherhood. Also make an agreement to practice with as little verbal language as possible, using signals and sound to communicate during your brotherly masturbation session. Agree to enjoy the animal intensity without ego games.

During such sessions, open your mind and heart to how the experience can re-connect you with your biological origins in Nature, as part of the Web of Life.

Cernunnos and the Green Man

In the centuries before the rise of the Roman Empire, the northern part of Europe was still largely continuous forest, though the inhabitants of the region were already in the process of deforesting some land for agriculture.

Many of the native tribes were pre-Celtic people with traditions more closely tied to Nature, including shamanistic and animistic beliefs and practices.

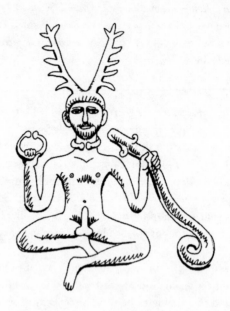

Cernunnos of the Forest

A woodland deity survived in these regions and times, a direct descendent or regional variation of Pançika, Shiva, Osiris, Pan, and Dionysus. Cernunnos, whose name apparently means something like "Horned God," or "The Horned One," was the male consort and partner with the Great Mother Goddess of the aboriginal European cultures that predated the Celts and the later Romans. Similar forms of the phallic, horned woodland god were known as Herne and Cruachan.

Cernunnos—sometimes called Lord of Animals, Lord of Wild Things, or the Great Horned One, and Lord of the Hunt—is a vibrant, yet non-violent fertility god of the woodlands. His image is of a mature, bearded man who sits cross-legged with the antlers of a stag upon his head. Around his neck he wears a torc or neck-ring of nobility, and sometimes he grasps a torc or torcs, or hangs them from his antlers.

He also wears wrapped about him, or grasps in his hands, the wondrous creatures called Horned Serpents—beings that signify natural wisdom, life force, and regenerative and lunar powers. These Horned Serpents are in fact European versions of the Sacred Cobras that Shiva wears around his neck and that often entwine his body. Like the early ithyphallic Mountain God images, Cernunnos sits fully erect. His phallus stands vertically upright as the World Axis and Tree of Life.

Cernunnos is the true male energy of the phallus, creative, physically strong and active, yet dynamic and peaceful because his phallic potency is integral with both his human and animal natures merged as One.

Among those aboriginal European tribes that long inhabited the vast forests of prehistoric Europe, another related male deity was the Spirit of the Great Oak, the Wildman or Green Man of the Woods. The Nordic people of the north venerated the World Axis in the form of their World Tree called Yggdrasil. Followers of the one-eyed Father God Odin hung sacrifices in the groves of sacred trees.

Like Osiris, who was sometimes described and shown as the Green God because of his connection with regenerative cycles of vegetative growth, and like Dionysus whose vegetative powers could cause ivy to suddenly grow like a wildfire, the Green Man exudes vitality and virility that sometimes challenges the constructed order of human civilization.

Though Osiris brought the civilized arts, his phallic nature as Menu-Osiris connected him with the phallic Valley God of vegetative powers. As a crossroads god, Osiris stood at the place where the living and the dead met. Dionysus fostered a kind of intoxicated wildness to temper the overly rational consequences of civilized cultures. Cernunnos and the Green Man similarly represented the pervasive potency of the vegetative intelligence. They also presided over the mysteries of life and death.

By some accounts, an actual cycle of sacred rule and annual sacrifice may have been practiced, in which a man was chosen to become King of the Wood for a year. Then this man sacrificed his predecessor to rule for the following year. At the end of the year the cycle repeated. This annual cycle aligns the traditions of the King of the Wood with other vegetative gods who die to be reborn.

Cycles of vegetative return, growth, abatement and regeneration likewise gave rise to the stories in which the King of Winter contended with the King of Summer for the love of the Maiden of Spring. Though to us, the outcome might seem inevitable, to tribal people this experience literally linked the enactment of certain rituals and mysteries with the cyclical progression of natural forces.

Such sympathetic magick not only encourages fruition, it also maintains the human connections with Nature.

As the Roman Empire gave way to the Church of Rome, which in a sense it *became* and then took over most of Europe, the Green Man remained popular. The peasant stone-carvers who helped to build the great churches and cathedrals assured that this Tree Spirit would persist; his male face peers out from many nooks and crannies, sprouting leaves in place of mustaches, beard, eyebrows and hair.

The phallic significance for you: Whether or not you are of European ancestry, the Horned God and Green Man of the aboriginal tribes of northern Europe speak to your DNA on the cellular level, for these later gods are directly related to Pan, Osiris, and Shiva.

While you masturbate mindfully, cultivate erotic energy or make love, relax and allow the ancestral awareness of such primordial Horned Gods, the Vegetative Phallic Lords of antiquity, to percolate from your unconscious into conscious awareness of your own body. While naked, place a pair of horns or antlers of some kind on your head, even part of a holiday costume. Masturbate while wearing this impressive headgear and observe yourself in a mirror while you masturbate. Abide with this image of yourself.

The New Millennium is a time when our species must reclaim our connection with the natural world, and create a green future for our descendants and ourselves.

Freyr: Phallic God of Pleasure and Peace

Near Uppsala in modern Sweden is the site of a large, major temple of the Norse phallic deity Freyr, known as the Lord of Pleasure and Peace, the Earth God, God of Summer and provider of both rain and sunshine…

Long, long ago two great families of gods, the Aesir and the Vanir are fighting a terrible war for domination of the world. The Aesir are heavenly warrior gods associated with the elements of air and fire and the sky Above. The Vanir are earthly fertility gods of water and earth and the surface world Below.

Among the Vanir, the Water God Njord is the first and oldest, and his twin sister, the Earth Goddess is called Nerthus. These primordial siblings unite as the elements of water and earth to feed the roots of the World Tree called Yggdrasil. Njord is also God of the Sea, patron of ships and seamen, of beaches and the seacoast, and all shoreline activities. His sacred bird is the seagull.

And so Njord takes Nerthus as his first wife. Such incestuous unions are quite common among the elder gods in almost every mythology.

From the mating of Njord and Nerthus is born another pair of twins, Freyr and his sister Freya. These siblings in turn serve as patrons of pleasure, fertility and abundance. Though Freya later takes on attributes of both love and war, her brother Freyr remains peaceable and non-violent, unless he is attacked or deeply offended.

At last the terrible conflict of the Aesir and the Vanir ends with a unification of the two tribes of gods. An amiable exchange of leaders formally concludes the hostilities, which is how Freyr and Freya come to live among the Aesir in their home at Asgard. There they flourish, and peace-loving Freyr is given the position of the highest ceremonial priest due to his skill in magickal arts. He reaches a status equaled only by Odin himself and his valiant son Thor.

An honor that the Aesir bestow upon Freyr is to give him rule over the realm of Alfheim or Elfland. The kingdom of Light Elves or nature spirits are those beings that tend to all of the living processes of Nature. Thus Freyr also comes to be called the Lord of Elves.

Freyr likewise has many incredible treasures that assist him on his adventures. These include the Golden Sword of Sunlight, not so much a weapon as a tool. It cannot fail in whatever he intends it to do, and he can use it to defend himself. Mostly his sword bestows the life-giving rays of the Sun. He also has the radiant golden-bristled boar Gullinbursti made for him by the dwarves, and a horse named Freyfaxi that can race across fire and air. Then there is a magickal ship called Skidbladnir, likewise a gift from the skillful dwarves, which can travel any direction regardless of the wind. Skidbladnir can bear a great army of men aboard it, and yet can also fold up to fit in Freyr's pocket.

All of these treasures represent aspects of Freyr's phallic powers as patron of the animating force behind all appearances of the natural world on the Earth. With these gifts and powers, Freyr governs the prosperity of men as well, and bestows upon them pleasure and peace.

He watches over farmers and gardeners and among his greatest gifts to the world are the beautiful flowers of forest and field. It is said that no weapon can be brought into his temples and no fighting should take place there. Though he has an earthly dwelling place where his great temple is built near Uppsala in Sweden, two other great temples of Freyr in ancient times are built at Throndhjein in Norway, and Thvera in Iceland.

His image is that of a handsome and virile bearded man, often shown with his sword and boar. A famous image of him shows a man sitting naked and cross-legged with a pointed hat and triangular beard that he pulls with one hand, while his huge phallus stands erect from his lap. In the "Ynglinga Saga" Snorri Sturlson describes the Norse gods as "men who came from India," so the resemblance of Freyr to Lord Shiva is not surprising. Even his extravagant mustaches resemble those of the early Mountain God images of the Indus Valley culture.

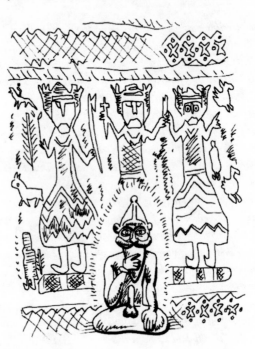

Freyr, Lord of Peace and Pleasure

A tapestry from 12ᵗʰ century Sweden even shows what appears to be Odin, Thor, and Freyr as a Norse version of the Triple God: Creator, Sustainer, and Regenerator.

Early tales tell of Freyr living at Uppsala as an actual king and the kings of Sweden later claim descent from him.

The phallic significance for you: Allow Freyr to remind you of your own deep connection with the Earth and how your ancestry has emerged like all else now living from common terrestrial ancestry. The full, shameless, and mindful embrace of your erotic potential holds the power of retroactive healing of ancient wounds, just as the war between the Aesir and Vanir ended in their unification.

In a real and essential sense all the male ancestors within you feel your pure penile pleasure and they share in your enjoyment. This also connects you on deep ancestral levels with all of humanity, just as the Norse gods are revealed to have connections with Pan and Shiva and all the powers of Earth and Sky. Freyr represents the qualities of authentic "masculinity" for he is strong, peaceful, playful and admirable.

Your penis has the same phallic powers represented by the treasures of Freyr: it is a phallic sword with life-giving solar qualities of male energy; your penis connects you with animal vitality, talents and fertility as with Freyr's magickal boar and magickal horse. His magickal ship, a phallic image because the shape and movement of a ship also suggests an erection, contains the "army" of male ancestors and can navigate or carry you wherever you will regardless of external factors such as "wind direction." Plus, though it has effects on a larger scale in the external arena of the world you live in, Like Skidbladnir your penis can be carried pocket-sized and concealed!

Regardless of your specific ancestry, accept Freyr as a divine inspiration.

You Stand at the Crossroads

Your phallus is literally your Source, and your inheritance from your male ancestors.

It's the origin of your life and the means to maintain yourself against the stress and stress and strain that can come with daily experience, as well as the means to transform yourself through constant regeneration, to reinforce your personal strengths, to drop weaknesses and to deal with the challenges you face in your daily life.

Of course, the creation of the world did not actually happen 13.7 billion years ago, or four thousand years ago; instead creation is ongoing in every moment. In the same way, whether aroused or not, on the deepest and highest levels your phallic regeneration occurs constantly.

The phallic energy, the same vertical, upward-moving current of sprouting, rising, growing, branching, leafing, flowering, that produces fruit and seed, and recycles the energy outward, back down and returns it inward below you to rise again through your form, is the energy of circulating life-force.

The male creative energy always operates while you live in a human male body. How effectively you deploy this energy is a factor of your attitude and awareness. The Secret of the Golden Phallus is that by cultivating this energy through Mindful Masturbation, Male Erotic Alchemy, and Golden Phallus Yoga you may increase and magnify its charge many times over and employ it to transform and regenerate yourself and determine the best path for your existence.

As you surrender to your inner potential and cultivate your embodied potency as a phallic god, you step onto the most natural and effective spiritual path for a human male.

Cultures and religions seek to keep this reality hidden from you simply because you will no longer need such external authorities or structures when you embrace and embark upon the Male Mysteries in your own experience and you become a Phallic Initiate. This does not mean you must deny or abandon your cultural or religious heritage, though there may be aspects of it that you will be required to seriously question.

To become a Phallic Initiate prepares you for the next step, to become a Phallic Adept, and possibly after that a Phallic Magus or Erotic Wizard.

These titles may sound occult and metaphysical, yet in practice they really involve no elaborate rituals or ceremonies, simply the direct experience and practice of masturbating mindfully. To advance through these initiations you learn the three forms of Male Solosex Magick, share Mindful Masturbation with fellow men to empower and energize the collective spiritual/erotic evolution of the Phallic Brotherhood of Men, and pursue your personal practice of Golden Phallus Yoga.

With this awareness you become the Herm at the crossroads of choice. You are the Valley God who is carried in procession in the Sacred Boat. You are the Lord of the Forest, Lord of Wild Animals, and the Green God.

This progression through the Male Mysteries is not theoretical, or symbolic, rather it's a natural and inevitable progression of experiential learning and development.

The Phallic Initiate is a man who wishes to access Phallic Wisdom from his own body; he pays full attention to the ancestral wisdom that emerges from his own cells. For this purpose he is willing to shift the focus of his erotic practice, at least temporarily, from partnered sex to Mindful Masturbation. The sole purpose of this shift is to keep his focus and preserve the charge of erotic energy he cultivates. He embraces solosexuality as a practice at least as valuable as any other form of sexual pleasure, and in fact more effective for a spiritual seeker until his third initiation into the Male Mysteries. He surrenders his limited sense of self in the process of becoming a phallic god. This man explores masturbating mindfully on a regular basis: solo, or in partnership, and in groups with Phallic Brothers.

The Phallic Adept is a man that practices Mindful Masturbation regularly, who consciously observes his own process, and deliberately breaks habitual patterns he detects in order to keep the doors of perception open. He pursues and practices the Three Forms of Male Solosex Magick. His erotic practice redeems and heals those male ancestors within him. He may choose to share the Male Mysteries of Mindful Masturbation with fellow men as a means of uplifting and empowering them and of refining and developing his own practice. The Adept may further choose to practice mutual Mindful Masturbation as a therapeutic form of conscious evolution and male bonding with Phallic Brothers.

The Phallic Magus or *Erotic Wizard* has consciously become a phallic god on a path of service to others, and awakened to that Oneness with All Things totally beyond words. This is experienced with awareness of his phallus as a spiritual umbilical that connects his body with Source. The Magus or Wizard learns directly from the cellular wisdom and the stardust of which his DNA is composed. He practices Golden Phallus Yoga, effortlessly and blissfully. He may choose to return to sharing other erotic practices such as oral, anal and vaginal sex with other people beyond the masturbatory path of the Initiate and the Adept, yet with a new level of self-confidence and ever-expanding awareness. He continues the endless learning of existence, yet only as divine play.

These three initiations into the Male Mysteries also correspond with the nature of the Triple God that is fully explained below, meaning the natural manner in which the threefold process of receiving, integration, and transmission unfolds in your life as an embodied human male.

When you feel totally alive and immortal in Penile Paradise, ironically you can also calmly face the mysteries of mortality. Full embodiment is the crossroads where living and dying become One process of ecstatic intensity beyond preferences, beyond likes and dislikes, beyond stories and personal drama. Ecstasy beyond understanding dissolves your ego. You no longer push away suffering or cling to pleasure.

Existence itself is a miraculous, magnificent, inexplicable gift.
The Great Mystery.

CHAPTER SIX:

YOU ARE THE TRIPLE GOD

Now is the time for men to reclaim our natural identification with the Great Phallic God just as so many women have reclaimed their natural connection with the Great Mother Goddess. In this sense women are ahead of men, as much knowledge and ritual has been reclaimed concerning the Triple Goddess in recent decades.

Less known until recently is the equally important Triple God, a major key to male self-awareness and empowerment.

The many phallic gods of various traditions are fathers, brothers, lovers and sons to the Maiden and the Mother and the Crone, as well as being fathers, brothers, lovers and sons to other male gods. The Triple God is not to be mistaken for those more recent Trinities of some current religions used to validate male dominance and competitive aggression during the last several millennia.

Rather, you must carefully discern those aspects of your authentic male creative energy that are not necessarily defined as "masculine," rather consider those that are innate to your biological reality as a male human.

Abstract symbols and concepts do not serve much purpose here. As the wise women of the new goddess culture explore experiential realities such as the power of sisterhood, the direct relation of menstruation to lunar cycles and to groups of empathetic women, motherhood, menopause, mature wisdom, and Wiccan circle work, so men are called to explore the Male Mysteries.

Men are designed and hard-wired as phallocentric creatures, a reality that the ancient Egyptians grasped literally and embraced in daily experience. All of the various mythic bits and pieces presented to you in this book converge in your own experience as you surrender to your inherent nature as a phallic god.

The original Trinity is the Holy Family, the Great Mother and the Good Father and their Holy Child.

Women have recovered the Triple Goddess: the Maiden, the Mother and the Crone. These relate to stages of life and progressive capacities potential in every female person.

Men must now reclaim the Triple God: the Youth, the Man, and the Sage.

As can you recognize, all three Trinities mentioned above represent actual human realities that are not theoretical, instead they are actual.

The Trinity of Three Trinities combined also provides an outline of eight archetypal human roles: Child, Maiden, Youth, Man, Mother, Father, Crone and Sage.

The Story of Dattatreya: the Triple God

The Divine Male Trinity of the Lords, the Creator, the Sustainer, and the Regenerator, has been venerated since the earliest Vedic times, perhaps 1500 BCE. More recently these three are called Brahma, Vishnu, and Shiva. You find evidence for the Triple God far earlier during the Indus Valley culture around 3000 BCE when the first known three-faced Mountain God image appears, and this archetypal Trinity may blend back into prehistory.

As the Creator, the Sustainer, and the Regenerator, these three major deities combined comprise the universal creative process. *All processes we know of can basically be described in terms of receiving energy, integrating or processing energy, and transmitting energy.* The three functions are aspects of a single universal process. Shiva carries a trident called the "Trishul" to signify this combined potency of Three in One Divinity, One in Three Divinities. Many of his devotees hold Shiva supreme and maintain that he embodies the whole Trinity.

Rather than wrestle with such concepts, however, simply consider these Triple Gods, this Divine Male Trinity as aspects of you.

The Creator is your youthful, playful, receptive aspect; the Sustainer is your manly, capable, responsible aspect; plus the Regenerator is your wise, beneficent, mature and sagacious aspect. These three are all parts of your wholeness as a human male. Though these aspects are most likely to unfold in a natural order with your experiences of living and growing and changing, all such potentials live within you all of the time.

An ancient story tells of how the Divine Male Trinity came to be incarnated in human forms as three brothers, and then how they merged into a single form called Dattatreya, or "Given to Seventh Son," for the sage named Atri, which means "Seventh Son," was Dattatreya's human father...

Long ago the great sage Atri lives in a forest hermitage with his devoted, pious wife called Anasuya, meaning "Free From Envy." They live a quiet life of meditation, in which they observe austerities and perform the traditional fire sacrifices. The famous divine sage Narada observes this ideal couple and during a visit with the Male Trinity of Brahma, Vishnu, and Shiva, he praises the virtues of Anasuya to the wives of the three great gods.

Though Narada has no such intention, his effusive praise of Anasuya causes the wives of the three great gods to grow jealous of her; so they ask their husbands to do something about this. "Please reduce Free From Envy's devotion to her husband Seventh Son," they ask, "so we will feel more comfortable when we hear about her."

Thus the Lords known as the Creator, the Sustainer, and the Regenerator assume appearances more like human mendicants begging for alms, rather than their awesome divine forms that sometimes appear with many arms, multiple faces and awesome auras.

When Atri is gone from home, the three gods disguised as hermits approach the forest hermitage to visit Anasuya.

"Oh Mother Anasuya! Give us some food," they say.

"Honored sages," she replies, "you are most welcome here! Yes, of course, please sit down and allow me to serve you."

"We are most grateful," Vishnu says, speaking for the Three. "However we will only accept the food if you agree to undress and serve us without any clothing on."

Anasuya lowers her gaze modestly. "Very well," she says softly. "I will do as you request." She goes to prepare the food for the three visitors, and when it is ready, she undresses and returns naked to serve them.

"Because you call me Mother," she says as she begins to serve the food, "I no longer view you as strangers, or as even as grown men. You are like my own children, very young and innocent. So I do not mind doing this for you."

The visitors eat the food and as they eat, due to the powers Anasuya's virtue has given her, their appearance changes from that of adult males to the appearance of small children. Upon sight of the three adorable little boys, she feels her breasts fill with milk, and the milk drops with her readiness to nurse them. So she nurses the three toddlers, and when they doze off with full stomachs, she places them in a hanging cradle, which she rocks slowly to help them sleep.

Before long, her husband Atri returns home. "Who are these beautiful babies?" he says in amazement, upon seeing the three. "And where did they come from?"

"They are honored guests," his wife says, "only I suspect that they are not what they appear to be! When they first arrived, they asked me to serve them their food only after I undressed. Someone has sent them to test me. I prayed to you, my husband, for guidance, and knew in my heart what you would say. I know that you trust my judgment.

"Now I realize that the Great Gods have generously given these three sons to a childless couple that has always longed for children of their own."

Upon hearing these words, the three babies awake and begin to cry, but when Anasuya lifts them from the cradle, they again begin to change and they assume their original immense and resplendent divine forms. Extra heads and arms appear, and resplendent auras emanate from their huge figures.

Of course, the pious couple falls down in worship before the Male Trinity as they appear in their splendid divine forms, with extra-human visages and limbs.

"Mother Free From Envy," Vishnu says, "you have shown admirable virtue and devotion to your husband, the noble sage Atri. What boon can we grant you? You have only to ask and it is yours."

Anasuya speaks humbly and presses her hands together before her heart, "Great Lords, my husband and I have no children of our own. I pray that we be given three sons, and because I have grown to love you as my own children, I ask that our sons be incarnations of you three."

"Granted," Vishnu says with a serene smile, and raises one of his four hands in an elegant mudra gesture of blessing.

Thus it comes about that Anasuya bears to her husband Atri three boys: Chandra, which means "Shining Moon" is an incarnation of the Creator Brahma, and he is also the Moon God. Dattatreya, meaning "Given to Seventh Son" is an incarnation of the Sustainer, Vishnu. Durvasa, or the "Impatient One" is an incarnation of the Regenerator, also known as Lord Shiva.

Eventually the three sons merge as the Triple God. They are even shown as a single body with three heads: the Creator, Sustainer, and Regenerator, from left to right. As such, this deity also becomes the first teacher of non-duality of the indescribable and inconceivable Oneness behind all apparent diversity and separation. As such, Dattatreya is a full incarnation in a single form of the Triple God.

The Triple God carries the Trishul, the Holy Trident of Shiva that has several levels of significance and a dog or dogs often accompany him. He embodies the three qualities of manifestation: purity, egotism, and darkness.

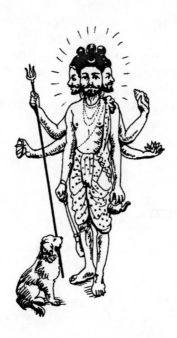

The Triple God: Dattatreya

Dattatreya makes major contributions to civilization. As a great scholar he becomes the first total master of the Four Vedas. He perfects the ritual use of the Elixir of the Gods, the Divine Nectar. By developing and refining the practice of Tantra, he achieves immense divine power and potency. His significance also merges the powerful austerities performed by his saintly father, Atri, and with the un-jealous and generous nature of his mother, Anasuya who is Free From Envy.

He's the One in Three; he's the Three in One!
The Triple God does not miss a thing!
He is all of your possibilities!

The phallic significance for you: Anytime you see a god that bears a trident, he's part of this Male Trinity. Though the details sometimes vary, the basic Male Trinity is within you. You are also in your deep essence this Triple God: the playful Youth, the responsible Man, and the wise Sage.

Embrace the gifts of your deepest genetic ancestry within the Tree of Life; let go of any stories of victimhood that you may inherit through personal history. Open your heart and mind to the highest or most expanded aspects of your ancestry, meaning the universal connections of your body's cells and molecules with stardust on the universal cosmic scale.

The Triple God by his attributes also reminds you of your own inherent close connection with the natural environment, with animal life, and the value of a spiritual perspective on worldly living. He makes clear that in a mysterious yet undeniable manner, Matter and Spirit are One…

Dance with this truth!

Trinity and Sacred Number

Many cultures—Eastern and Western—contain an extremely simple, yet subtle and profound teaching about what is called Sacred Number. In essence this is precisely the same truth. Sacred Number comprises the very simplest and subtlest model of how the world comes into being, and as such relates directly to your own sacred phallus as the singular generator of your male creative energy.

The Taoist sage Lao Tzu said:

"Out of nothing comes the One;
Out of One comes the Two;
Out of Two comes the Three;
Out of Three comes All Things."

The Egyptian teaching of Sacred Number likewise tells the Creation Story, or portrays the essential creative process in virtually identical terms. As such, "number" is not about quantity or counting. Rather, Sacred Number refers to qualities, processes and relationships that are more actual than the separate things that are related.

Thus:

One is absolute, indivisible Unity.

Two is Duality, arising as self-reflection within unity.

Three is Trinity, which arises simultaneously with Duality, as the relationship between the Two that returns the Duality back into Oneness. (Sometimes this relationship is called Love.) *Remember the three eyes of Lord Shiva; the two Below echo his testicles, while the vertical Third Eye Above stands for his erect penis.*

The triangular principle of the process of Sacred Trinity actually does nothing to compromise the absolute, indivisible unity of One.

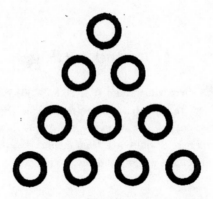

Tetractys: The Inner Dynamic of Creation

Still, the Three enact the unseen, inner dynamic of Creation that facilitates emergence of the Sacred Number Four. The image of ten points arranged in a triangle, called the "Tetractys," illustrates this dynamic described by the Pythagorean mystics of ancient Greece. Pythagoras is said to have learned about it in Egypt.

Four is the elements of manifest physical reality: Earth, Water, Air, and Fire.

The first Three are all the numbers you need to describe the dynamic process of creation—and Four are all the fourfold markers of visible and material experience, such as the four directions, the seasons, the major times of day, and so on.

As such, *all* numbers are sacred!

All mythologies of every culture in the world can be understood from the inside-out with this basic awareness of Sacred Number and how it relates to the three basic trinities: the Holy Family, the Triple Goddess, and the Triple God.

You need not learn the amazing and extremely complex hieroglyphic language of the ancient Egyptians in order to make sense of their complex artworks and artifacts.

All of these levels ultimately return back into the One, which corresponds with your phallus as the organ that generates pleasure capable of connecting you in Oneness with All Things.

The Youth, the Man, and the Sage

For men of this New Millennium (CE 2000-3000) it helps to reclaim awareness of the Triple God, as women reclaim the Triple Goddess. The three stages or forms of divinity are more than simply those inevitable ages of a lifetime: from birth to adulthood, from manhood to the maturity of an elder, and the final years of wisdom and perspective.

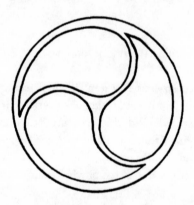

Three in One; One in Three

The Triple God is the full range of your divine attributes as a phallic god embodied in human form. The Triple God expresses essential divinity through you as you experience the stages of personal development inherent to the human male you are. The Triple God in all of his forms is phallic in nature and biologically male.

The Triple God also brings to you the inheritance from your ancestors.

These Three are not stages you pass through and leave, any more than the Unity of One, the Duality of Two, and the Trinity of Three are separate qualities. Rather the Three form a dynamic process. They co-exist as qualities of the male creative energy, always present within you at least as potentials.

Youth and Young Manhood

Western cultures in particular are in hysterical denial concerning the sexuality of children. In fact, prenatal ultrasound imagery reveals that boys sometimes begin to masturbate before birth. Humans are highly sexual creatures from the beginning.

In fact, many baby boys are born with an erection and may have orgasms shortly after birth. The truth is, as midwives sometimes testify and doctors seldom wish to discuss at all, it is quite natural and often desirable for a woman in the labor of delivery to actually have orgasms while she gives birth. Between the rounds of painful contractions, a mother in labor may be well advised to masturbate or accept stimulus from helpers. This assists with her pain and increases the ease of delivery.

Doubtless the child that is still part of the mother in the most literal sense also feels her ecstatic sensations that mix with the pain of the ordeal for both child and mother.

Of course as newborn boy you could not ejaculate until at least another eleven, twelve or thirteen years had passed. Yet all along you may have erections, and experience orgasms or states of orgasmic intensity. By age five or six, you may have discovered masturbation for yourself, or at least found out how good it feels to exert pressure between your legs when aroused! Genital play or the enjoyment of pressure between the legs is something that as a boy you may not have associated consciously with any clear awareness of sexuality. Yet you knew it felt great!

Many good-intentioned parents and guardians feel uncomfortable when they observe such behavior and seek to inhibit or control this kind of activity. Such interventions can lead to problems of lack of confidence, poor self-esteem, and general shame over sexuality during the transition from childhood into the teens and early adulthood. This can even last a lifetime.

Most important for you now is to reclaim your Original Innocence, even if you suffered some of the common challenges from the earliest age, at the core of your being is the inner child. No matter how deep inside this child may be, he is there, intact, pure and perfect!

You need not indulge in nostalgic fantasy to recover the deepest essence of your erotic nature that remains free from uncertainty, fear, ego-games and the need for approval. The child within you knows what feels good and knows that it *is* good. As this child, you love yourself naturally; you are not confused by ideas that come from others. In your heart you know what is right and good.

By the time you grow up it is easy to forget, or enter into denial about how intensely you experienced erotic energy as a child. The mere idea of nakedness or genitals often proves almost intolerably exciting to a young child. The classic scenarios of "playing doctor," or playing "Adam and Eve," may satisfy curiosity.

When you entered adolescence you probably discovered how important it was to claim some private space in order to explore the changes you were experiencing.

The best antidote to the unrealistic abomination of "abstinence" teachings is to encourage young men to develop masturbatory excellence. Young men should also be encouraged to masturbate together, which is safe and can be as deeply rewarding as any form of sex. Young men should be encouraged not to label themselves according to limited prefab identities of the old paradigm such as "gay," "bisexual," or "straight." How about "intensely sexual human male"?

When you accept 100% responsibility for everything that shows up in your reality because you somehow participate in its creation, you can no longer be the victim of anyone or anything else outside of you. When you honor and value masturbation at least as much as any other erotic activity, you accept 100% responsibility for your own pleasure. In reality, nothing is more pure and innocent than male masturbation.

Not only is it possible to regain your Original Innocence; also, *as you read these words, you are already on your way there!* You will learn how to redeploy your erotic energy to lift old imprints and to re-imprint a happier, healthier, more balanced reality.

To replace the past with ongoing, magnificent experiences of erotic ecstasy in the present, here and now, is the key.

Mature Manhood

For a boy in his teens, with the physical maturation of the body comes a stunning revelation of how extremely powerful erotic sensations can be! Not only has the body increased in size and strength, with such secondary sexual characteristics as body hair and a lower voice, but the increased size and sensitivity of the penis and testicles, and perhaps the nipples as well, all become amazing realms of discovery.

Older men, often distracted by all sorts of other personal, social and professional concerns, easily forget the wonder and amazement that attends the new experiences that become possible with puberty.

During your teens, you physically leave the planet of childhood. Only much later do you have the opportunity to recognize this for what it is: the literal emergence of your male ancestry within your body. During adolescence, emotions, sensations, and thoughts all become amplified in intensity.

For the sake of humanity and the planet *it is crucial that we institute a new matricentrist culture.* This means a genuine partnership of the sexes, in which the values of motherhood and female choice are not only protected, but also considered sacrosanct. Reproductive responsibility must be taken seriously on our over-populated planet. Also, females must be relieved of unwelcome sexual attention and allowed to select their mates without coercion. Women must emerge into more and more positions of authority. In historical terms, a realistic view reveals that this is our only hope as a species.

For purely erotic and physical pleasures mature males must also be actively encouraged to pursue both excellence in solosexuality and to seek same-sex playmates for masturbatory and other forms of erotic sharing.

We already live on a New Earth.

The "nuclear family" as now defined and monogamous marriage are actually quite recent inventions. Of course, some female/male partnerships do prove to be extremely rewarding, and enduring for both partners. However, given the false conditioning about "masculinity" and "femininity" that pervades the old paradigms, which persist in many people's minds, such a partnership often proves challenging.

A monogamous, totally exclusive partnership with the expectation of lifelong fidelity to one person who is expected to be all things to you, is seldom realistic for humans. For emotionally mature and responsible adults of all kinds, a sort of polyfidelity of committed, open and honest relationships with several people, possibly of both sexes, may work better than the traditional model of monogamous marriage.

Perhaps this still seems shocking to many, and yet it is the truth of human nature. In most tribal and hunter-gatherer cultures such polyfidelity tends to be the norm more than monogamous marriage, which is quite rare. Children benefit from the nurturing and care of an extended family beyond their biological parents.

Mature manhood of today involves not only responsible fatherhood and parenting, but also being a brother and mentor, and friend who can encourage the best in others.

The New Earth is about exploring many possibilities.

Wisdom

In traditions worldwide, the shaman, sage or wise elder (though he is not always old) is sometimes called the "wounded healer." The wound means that he has suffered greatly and the healer means that he has healed himself. This provides him with wisdom and insight into the fact that mortality is a mystery and that life is for the living to embrace with gratitude.

The wounded healer also connects this third aspect of the Triple God with the Green Man and hence Osiris, who was sometimes called the Green God. The green is that vegetative force of the rising, vertical, phallic energy. Whether Osiris literally died or not, he "healed" himself and was resurrected through an act of sacred masturbation, as described here in more detail later on. The phallic power of loving himself intensely enough, with enough passion brought him back to life.

As the Sage you come home to a happier childhood than your first one, even if you were happy then! Your natural home is Paradise, as you recognize this is actually H.O.M.E.—meaning Humanity's One Mother Earth. H.O.M.E.

The mainstream media still holds many people in the grip of its cultural trance, though it continues to broadcast from the dead old paradigm. Those who believe what the mainstream media tells them about the world and about life are likely to struggle with toxic negativity, pessimism and despair. Through that shadowy lens it's almost impossible to recognize the truth of what is happening, which is challenge and opportunity.

The Old Earth is a hopeless, apocalyptic place, in which humanity remains suicidally addicted to fossil fuels, gripped by insatiable consumer/ shopping psychosis, and in the thrall of an irresistible War Machine funded by the corporate hegemony that has taken over all political systems of the planet. The growth at any cost mandates of the past have become simply unsustainable.

Fortunately the Old Earth is now only a story, a set of false assumptions and beliefs that, like 99% of all your beliefs and everyone's beliefs, has no actual validity.

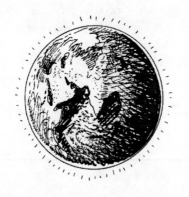

Gaia

On the New Earth the primary paradigm is Love and it begins with loving yourself better and better, as best you are able.

Planet Earth is evolving rapidly.

The Global Brain is smarter than its parts.

Gaia is very much alive and continues to provide everything its children need.

We now face our most crucial and exciting choices as a species. The only viable option for a good future is to make peace with ourselves, with each other, and with the natural world. We cannot accomplish this until we reclaim a healthy relationship with our bodies and our erotic energy. These issues are bound up together. There is always a direct correspondence between what happens to the individual person and what happens to the planet.

The Sage is a man who has fully experienced adulthood and sees it for what it is, merely an episode in his journey of return to the essence of who and what he has been all along. ***Much of the growth process of adulthood is to shed the acquired layers of who and what you are not!*** After all, the word "adult" means literally "an organism that has stopped growing," so as your growth continues, this label too must be shed.

Peter Pan refused to grow up because he had never lost that Original Innocence that the Sage reclaims. The Sage looks deep within himself, to recover his inherent authenticity. He also regains his childlike curiosity, sense of wonder, and enthusiasm, a sincere playfulness and spontaneity.

What a relief to admit that you know almost nothing, that wisdom, which proceeds from the heart, matters far more than acquired information!

The Sage looks into the eyes of death and does not flinch, even if his heart breaks. He does what he knows in his heart is right for the sake of the living and the dead. He sees the mystery that cannot be spoken, despite the following words…

Life and death are not what we have imagined them to be.

They are not separate or even different.

They are One.

CHAPTER SEVEN:

THE ITHYPHALLIC RESURRECTION

You have come this far into the Male Mysteries, my Brother; it is now too late to turn back. You will never be the same man you were before, which in many ways is something to be grateful for.

Each time your penis grows erect and rewards you for stimulating its pleasure receptor nerves, you return from whatever else you experienced to this condition of feeling intensely alive and progressively regenerated. Male Erotic Alchemy allows you to experience prolonged states of orgasmic bliss, or even multiple orgasms, without the interruption of an ejaculatory orgasm followed by a refractory period before your enjoyment can resume.

Great mindful masturbators often report a state in which nothing seems to exist except for the penis. *"It's all nothing but One Big Penis!!!"* Here the common mind and body separation that is so often the human condition collapses back into the continuum of the unconditioned, a genuine taste of Oneness.

Everything alive is in the process of dying; everything dying is in the process of living. So are these different processes? Or are they aspects of a far more mysterious reality that cannot be described in words?

Just as the process of creation continues all the time, you were not actually born on the day of your birth: you are being born now, with every breath you take, with each beat of your heart, with every nanosecond that you exist.

In ancient Egypt the Good God Osiris had to die in order to become the Great God Osiris. Before he died he was King of the Living, Lord of the Two Lands of Egypt, described as Forever Young. As the Great God he became King of Eternity, Lord of Souls, and Lord of Silence.

But was this "death" necessarily the actual destruction of his biological form? It can be understood as "dying" to the stress and strain of ordinary everyday life in order to evolve into a new state of existence. It can mean dying to the limited sense of the individual human self to unite with the Great Self of the Universe.

Both of these interpretations perfectly describe what you experience when you grow aroused and erect, and you generate erotic ecstasy of sufficient quality and duration to alter your consciousness from the mundane to the magnificent.

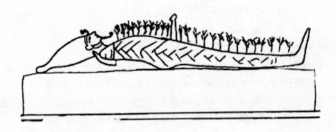

The Green God as the Vegetative Power of Growth

Likewise keep in mind that Osiris is the Green God; like the later European Green Man, he is a natural deity of the vegetative cycles of germination, growth, dying and regeneration. Each year the ancient Egyptians made images of the slain god from soft clay mixed with seeds, to be watered so the whole thing sprouted to demonstrate the phallic god's return from the seed state.

You are able to naturally alter your brain chemistry and hormones safely and effectively through Mindful Masturbation and Male Erotic Alchemy in order to bring about permanent changes for the better in the quality of your experience of living.

Resurrection is this regenerative power, to let go of the old way of living and to be born anew with every moment, with each breath, every beat of your heart, with each pulsation of your penis.

The Golden Phallus

*O*siris and Isis simply appear from the East, walk into the Nile Valley of Egypt, and they become the first Divine Couple to rule the Two Lands. This Lord and Lady bring all the arts and knowledge of civilization with them, and they build the first city. With them come their sister, Nephthys, and their brother called Set.

Nephthys, the Lady of the House, is married to Set the Hunter. He pursues a primitive way of life, hunting in the marshy reed inlets along the river. Though she is married to Set, Nephthys prefers the company of Isis and Osiris. She spends much of her time with them and presides in their home as Lady of the House. While Isis is gone, Nephthys impersonates her sister, gets Osiris drunk and sleeps with him. When she bears a son, his name is called Anubis, and his actual father is Lord Osiris, not Set.

Set is already envious of Osiris and Isis and their kingdom, the Two Lands, whose people adore and worship them, and when he learns that Osiris is the father of Anubis, he devises an evil plot for revenge. He invites Osiris to share a fine banquet with him, without their wives present. Though Isis and Nephthys are suspicious, Osiris insists on going alone. He says, "It is a sign of trust."

After they share the good food and plenty of drink, Set shows his brother a beautiful box, made precisely to fit the size and shape of Osiris's body. "Oh, let me see if it fits me as it appears to," Osiris says trustingly.

"Let me help you try it out," Set says and gives his brother a hand, as Osiris steps into the box and lies down. Immediately the followers of Set rush in, stab Osiris to death and seal the box, which becomes his coffin. They cast it into the Nile, where it floats downstream, through the delta and onto the northern sea.

Isis quickly discovers what has happened. Through her powers and arts, she finally retrieves the body of her slain husband. Once she has returned the body home, Set discovers this. "If we don't do something drastic," he tells his minions, "Isis will try to bring him back to life!" So they sneak into the place where Isis keeps the coffin, and cut the body of Osiris into fourteen parts. "Now scatter these pieces far and wide," Set tells them and they obey.

Regardless, Isis eventually manages to find all the pieces, except for the phallus of Osiris, which has been thrown into the river and eaten by a fish called the Abtu fish.

Undaunted, Isis reassembles the thirteen pieces that still exist. In order to facilitate the resurrection of her husband, Isis fashions a golden phallus and attaches it to the reassembled body of Osiris. She knows that she alone cannot bring him back to life—she can only make it possible for him to re-animate himself through an act of sacred masturbation.

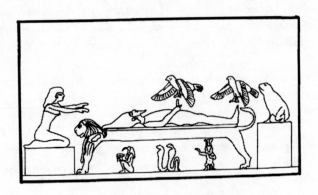

The Osiris Bed

Egyptian vignettes commonly called "The Osiris Bed" depict the masturbatory self-reanimation of Osiris. He is seen lying on his back on the funerary couch, which has the shape of a lion. He masturbates his golden phallus in order to bring himself back to life. A frog of fertility that is the goddess Heqt stands at his feet. The Lady of the West, the goddess Hathor, who welcomes souls into the Western Lands, kneels at his head.

In the process of resurrecting himself, Osiris spiritually conceives his son, Horus, in the soul bird of Isis. Osiris rises, but he is transformed and becomes the Lord of Souls and King of Eternity who rules in the Western Lands. Later, his son Horus is born to rule as Lord of the Living, and father and son are closely identified and serve the same purpose for the Living and for the Dead.

They are the Son and the Father of All Things.

The phallic significance for you: The Golden Phallus is the power of regeneration that you inherit from your male ancestors. This is not literally about death, rather this concerns restoration from the shattering and deadly aspects of daily living. Use your innate phallic power to regenerate yourself.

The erection of your penis now becomes the alchemical gold created by the philosopher's stone, that "Midas touch" of expanded consciousness, which dissolves the everyday world of familiar habit and limiting beliefs. It renders every moment of your existence miraculous and precious beyond measure. To live in the present moment becomes an amazing adventure without beginning or end.

The Golden Phallus is your power to transform your consciousness at every moment by touching your own body and manipulating your penis, to expand your awareness beyond words.

The Vibrant Life of Egyptian Imagery

A major hieroglyph for "phallus" in ancient Egyptian simply shows a horizontal erection from the side, head on the left and balls on the right, as if the erect man stands up, facing left. A small curved line to the left of the glans indicates ejaculation emerging and falling. Pronounced "met" according to standard English phonetics, it means "phallus, front, male, masculine, or procreate."

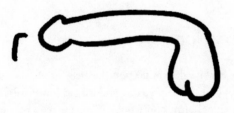

Egyptian Hieroglyph for "Phallus"

As you can see, the glyph is naturalistic, with nothing abstract or metaphorical about it. For the male Egyptian, this glyph had all of the energy, immediacy and actuality of the organ rooted between his own legs. There were at least nine major terms for the phallus in ancient Egypt, most of which had quite a few variations. Thus as the Inuit language has many specific terms for snow, the Egyptian language offers numerous nuances having to do with the erect penis.

The web of associations includes the actions "to present," "to rise," "to offer," "to beget," "to copulate," "seed," "beauty," plus the youthful trinity of "child, youth, young man," among other phallic nuances.

Later people have often misunderstood the purpose of sacred images in many ancient cultures including Egypt. What later Western culture calls idolatry or idol worship was never worship of the image itself, rather the ancients honored and venerated the vital presence that inhabited the image by invitation. Egyptian sacred images were in fact "brought to life" by a ritual in which the actual presence of the deity represented was petitioned and invited to enter into and inhabit the image. For the ancients, the images actually lived.

In the temple, the faithful could *see* the gods themselves in the Living Images.

The phallic significance for you: Regardless of your sexuality, you can experience something of how imagery holds a potent vital charge of presence by meditation upon any explicit or erotic image that especially turns you on. Notice how your fascination and arousal by the imagery kindles actual sensations of aliveness in your own body. This is not necessarily idolatry, rather it can be seen as a connection in which boundaries dissolve.

Penis Reflexology 101

Thoroughly explore the connections between your penis and the rest of your whole body to help you to understand how Osiris brings himself back to life by an act of masturbation. Whenever you thoroughly massage your penis from its root to the crown at the tip of the head, if you remain relaxed and breathing deeply into your belly, the tonic benefits of your pleasurable sensations permeate all the rest of you from the soles of your feet to the crown of your head.

One way to understand this holistic quality of masturbating mindfully is through Penis Reflexology. Reflexology in general is a treatment and healing process based on the fact that everything in the body is connected with everything else. Both Oriental Medicine and modern massage therapies make use of the concept that specific locations on the feet, the hands and the ears correspond with all other portions of the body as a whole.

Though the medical establishment remains skeptical of the effectiveness of reflexology, this practice originates from China perhaps 5000 years in the past, and a form of reflexology was also practiced in ancient Egypt. Now, often termed "alternative medicine," in reality this is a matter of "whatever works." For example, the benefits of foot massage are well known and practiced worldwide.

By massaging and manipulating specific points and areas on a foot, a hand, or an ear, you connect with specific corresponding organs or other areas of the body. Each foot, hand or ear definitely contains concentrations of sensitive nerve endings that ultimately connect with the entire body through the central nervous system of spine and brain, so this makes sense.

Your magnificent, highly evolved human penis with its concentrations of sensitive nerve endings can also be understood in terms of reflexology, with specific locations that correspond and connect with other specific regions of your body as a whole.

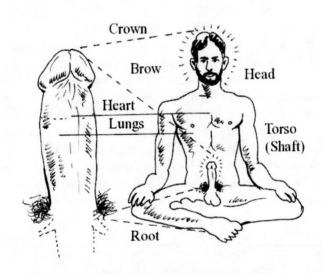

Penis Reflexology

The correspondences depicted here are connections you are encouraged to experiment with, play with, and test for yourself. The more thoroughly you stimulate your aroused genitalia, the more rewarding your erotic ecstasy proves to your entire body. So consider your penis, as mentioned before, as a microcosm of your entire body; and your entire body is a macrocosm of your penis.

From Root to Crown: The roots of your penis are actually like a tripod that supports its "draw-bridge" function of erection. The two firmer inner chambers (the *Corpora cavernosa*) along the upper sides of the shaft have smaller roots anchored into your inner thighs; the main spongy inner chamber (*Corpus spongiosum*) has an internal root that passes back through your perineum almost to your anus. These roots of your penis correspond and connect with your anus and the sacrum that lies at the base of your spine, all of which "grounds" you as you sit.

The shaft of your penis as a whole corresponds and connects with your torso as a whole, just as the head of your penis corresponds with the head on your shoulders. Those two firmer chambers within the shaft that run its length from the base to the beginning of the head, correspond with your ribcage and lungs.

The longer spongy inner chamber that contains the urethra passage for both urination and ejaculation of semen corresponds to and connects with your spinal column and brain. The outer or upper end of this spongy chamber flares out to form the resilient inner mass of your mushroom head—the acorn shape of your glans—and this bulbous shape can be considered the "brain" of your penis.

If you are intact, the location on the underside of the shaft where your foreskin attaches corresponds and connects with your heart. For circumcised men this location on the penis lies where the circumcision scar crosses the middle of the underside below the head. This connection lies close to the *frenulum* at the underside of the glans itself, which for many men is extremely sensitive.

This frenulum, from a Latin term that means "bridle," as in a horse's bridle, correspond and connects with your brow, or what yogis call the Third Eye center of intuition, inner sight and visionary insight.

The tip of your penis, where the meatus (from the Latin for "passage"), the opening of the urethra at the end of the glans, is located, corresponds and connects with the sagittal suture at the crown of your cranium or the tip-top of your skull. Just as the meatus is a location where precum (Cowper's gland secretion) may emerge for some men during high arousal as clear droplets of slick fluid, the top of the head is a place yogis call the Crown Chakra or "Thousand-Petalled Lotus."

As such, the crown is considered a place of connection with the universal totality, which occurs when you begin to generate the Divine Nectar within your brain.

Male Mysteries of the Osiris Bed

Every night when you go to sleep your conscious awareness dissolves and seems to go away totally. You become unaware of your everyday waking reality, and experience either dream sleep or dreamless oblivion. In one sense, this is a daily "little death." All too easily we take the return from that "void" state for granted.

Likewise for human males, the testosterone cycle of your body tends to peak sometime in the early morning hours and may inspire night erections. Men sometimes call early erections "morning wood." Such erections can provide especially delicious, glorious sensations when you choose to pleasure yourself in that wonderful twilight state between sleep and wakefulness.

What is perhaps the most famous story in the world, that of the Goddess and her consort the Dying God who is resurrected (and its many variations in other cultures) relates directly to this matter of nighttime erections. In fact, if you are a human male beyond puberty the story is entirely about *you*. The stress and strain of daily living may fragment you, and to treat your penis as the Golden Phallus has the power to regenerate all of you and restore you to your innate wholeness.

The crucial juncture of the story of Isis and Osiris is when she presides at the resurrection of her slain husband from the dead. A common version of the story credits Isis not only with re-assembling the body of her slain husband, but also with his resurrection. While she certainly put his pieces back together, another telling credits the god himself with his actual resurrection. He is responsible for his regeneration. Osiris accomplishes this by an act of masturbation.

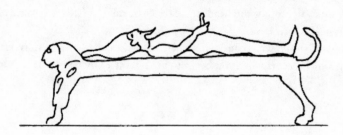

Osiris Resurrecting Himself

The Good God lies on his back on a "lion-bed" or lion-shaped funerary couch. His head rests on the end closer to the lion's front legs and the head end of the couch, while his feet lie upon its hind legs and tail end. The erect lion tail curves upward and points in the same direction as the flow of energy through the god's body from his feet to his head.

The god's penis is erect and he grasps his phallus in his hand in the act of masturbation, a practice for which the Egyptians had at least seven basic terms. He performs a sacred masturbatory ritual that is alchemical, because he is "dead" and it will transform him from merely a "Good God" into a "Great God," and restore him to life, health and strength. After his "resurrection" Osiris passes into the Western Lands to rule as the Lord of Souls, while his son Horus, magickally conceived within Isis by this process, is destined to rule in his name over the Living.

Alchemy is this Great Work of transformation and regeneration.

To masturbate in this manner can bring you back to life from the ways in which daily existence has diminished you and scattered you into fragments; your parts have been scattered in separated disunity. Most extremely of all, your phallus has been lost from all the rest of you by beliefs that it must be kept hidden and must not be seen.

This really is not about a mythic god who may have lived as an actual king four or five millennia in the past in Egypt. This is about you now, and the power that a total surrender to erotic ecstasy has for you to transform and regenerate yourself every day.

Let's explore a particular Osiris Bed vignette that has special significance for every man interested in practicing Male Erotic Alchemy.

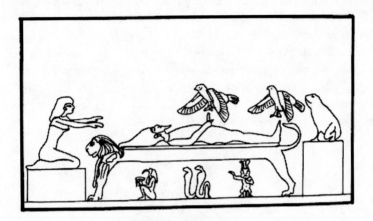

Details of the Osiris Bed

Seven deities surround the figure of Osiris on the lion-bed of his golden, solar, male energy. These seven generally resemble the seven chakras, or energy-centers of Yoga that has roots in the Indus Valley culture, so this vignette suggests a certain congruence between the two great civilizations.

Place yourself in the image as Osiris. The seven Egyptian gods are arranged around your body in a manner that depicts the flow of what yogis call Serpent Fire. This is the life force, the universal creative energy as it manifests in your human body.

You lie in the Yoga position called "Corpse Pose," relaxed and flat on your back, with this variation: hold your erect penis in your hand.

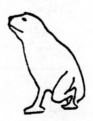

Heqt as Abundant Energy

Below your feet is the living image of a frog, which is also the goddess *Heqt*, the patron of waters. She presides over the birth of all creatures. Here she sits up alert, and lively, in the form of a huge frog. She represents your literal connection with the ground beneath your feet. Heqt is associated with the east, the place light comes from at each daybreak. She is the prolific energy of spawning, producing numberless eggs and tadpoles, and represents tremendous natural abundance. Heqt sends a powerful current of living energy upward from your feet through your body.

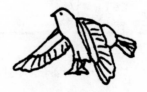

The Soul-Bird of Nephthys, Lady of the House

Nephthys is seen hovering over your feet in the form of a soul-bird, which appears as a little hawk in flight. The bird faces the direction in which the energy flows in your body, from feet to head. The energy rises through you. Nephthys is those domestic, nurturing qualities that comfort and protect you, which you stand upon. Nephthys makes you feel secure and safe enough to claim your own private personal space.

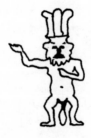

Bes, the Dwarf God of Happiness, Friend of Women

Beneath the lion-bed stand three deities. The first of these in order is *Bes*, the bringer of happiness, patron of music and friend of women. Bes is a Nubian dwarf, both jolly and fierce. He is a loyal guardian and also the life of every party. His huge phallus (though some mistakenly call it a lion's tail) hangs all the way to the ground! He stands below your calves and knees, important when you walk or dance. A humorous character and a god that encourages dancing, Bes is shown touching his heart with one hand, with the other hand lifted open in a reminder of blessings and gratitude for blessings.

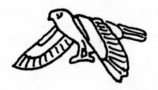

The Soul-Bird of Isis, Mistress of Enchantments

Isis herself, in the form of another soul-bird, a small falcon identical with that of her sister Nephthys, hovers over your phallus. The Beautiful One, Mistress of Enchantments, Goddess of Goddesses who is the Soul of the Universe, Lady Isis reminds you of the power of hovering indefinitely in high arousal. Retain your semen while you continually stimulate your erect penis with artful awareness and skilled intensity. Pursued diligently, this can change you forever.

Isis hovers directly above your erection to remind you that it is she who has replaced your "missing" penis with the Golden Phallus and makes this Magick possible.

Together the two soul-birds of the sisters of Osiris suggest the fluttering, whirring, delicate and feathery artfulness of your caresses to your erect penis during skilled, artful, mindful self-pleasure.

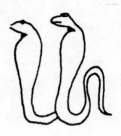

The Two Serpents of Power

The Two Serpents, or Solar Cobras, below the lion-bed under the lower back of Osiris travel without moving. While you masturbate mindfully they undulate in place along your spine, and carry signals between your genitals and your brain. Yogis call this the Serpent Power, and label the two waves of energy the "ida" and the "pingala." They name the pathway that corresponds with the spine overall, the "shushumna." In the Vedic culture that followed the Indus people, the Lord Sustainer Vishnu reclines on the back of this Cosmic Serpent that floats in the Ocean of Milky Bliss.

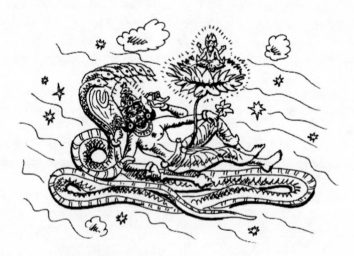

The Sustainer Vishnu on the Cosmic Serpent

This is not theoretical! Your sensations arise from the constant two-way traffic of central nervous system signals along the spine between genitals and brain. A continuous feedback circuit that travels both ways becomes self-reinforcing as a kind of constructive wave interference and amplifies your sensations. You alter your consciousness and you evolve.

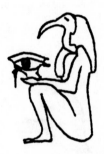

Lord Tehuti, God of Wisdom

Tehuti sits beneath the headrest of your lion-bed. He appears in this vignette as a seated male figure with the head of a sacred ibis. His wrists rest on his knees and in both hands he holds the Wisdom Eye of Atum. In yogic tradition this Eye is the Third Eye, or the brow center. Tehuti is also a Phallic Moon God, Scribe of the Gods, Inventor of Language and Master of Magick: the God of Wisdom.

Just as the ibis stalks the shallows, to dip its beak into the water and there it finds things to eat, the Third Eye helps you to clearly *see* the unseen. Sometimes Tehuti is depicted as an old man, which relates him to the Sage or third aspect of the Triple God.

Your heart naturally begins to soften and open with the Serpent Power that flows along your spine both ways between genitals and brain. This heart opening does not mean romantic love or even emotional attachment, so much as a deeper and higher, more fearless and open connection with existence itself.

The Wisdom Eye is your inner vision, the intuitive knowing—sometimes called a gut feeling or instinct—that does not depend on external information. It comes from deep within you. Within you is everything you may experience *as if* it was outside of your body and yourself. *It is all really happening inside of your body, where you create images of what seems to be outside of your body.*

In reality everything IS happening within you.

When you consciously accept 100% responsibility for how much erotic pleasure you experience, and also 100% responsibility for the quality of your ecstasy, you achieve a remarkable kind of freedom. This is how you actually become a phallic god.

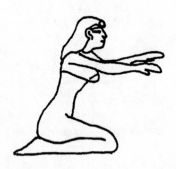

Hathor, Lady of the West, Golden Lady

Above your head facing you on her knees with both hands extended in blessings upon you is Hathor, the Lady of the West, whose name means "House of the Face," or "House of the Falcon." This face is *your* face as the Falcon Prince, the divine heir of all your male ancestors: the King of your Life.

Hathor is the maternal, eternal aspect of Isis.

The ultimately gracious hostess, Hathor welcomes the Sun Boat into its evening harbor with every nightfall. She also welcomes souls of the Dead through her doorway into the Western Lands. Hathor is the western complement to the eastern Heqt, as they are stationed at the head and foot of the lion-bed respectively.

The flow of living energy is a continuous cycle, without end or beginning.

Some things about human nature, in essence, have not changed for millennia. This is why the cellular memories triggered by your erotic practice connect directly with these mythic images from the human past. In ancient

Egyptian terms, this is the process of Male Erotic Alchemy for the 21st Century:

- **Heqt unleashes the powerful vital force through your body, root-to-crown.**

- **Nephthys provides a secure and stable foundation to stand on.**

- **Bes inspires celebration, dancing, music, and stirs phallic energy.**

- **Isis presides over your cultivation of erotic energy as the male creative, sustaining and regenerative power with the Golden Phallus.**

- **The Two Serpents carry this phallic Serpent Fire along its Royal Road.**

- **The Wisdom Eye opens as Tehuti appears at your brow.**

- **Hathor gestures from above the crown of your head, to recycle all of the energy back through the entire system.**

Similarly the Sun Boat of Ra moves in an endless cycle, westward over the world and back east through the Underworld. This is the flow of erotic energy through your body as you cultivate your high and sustained charge.

You practice artful, creative self-pleasure as a means of loving yourself…

You are doing it: ***Male Erotic Alchemy for the 21st Century!***

Every Erection is a Resurrection

There are no limits to the depths and heights to which Male Erotic Alchemy can take you. The deepest depths are within your body, inside the molecules of your ancestral DNA, and within the matter/energy of your stardust.

An alchemical teaching attributed to Hermes Trismegistus says: "As Above, so Below. As Below, so Above. As Without, so Within. As Within, so Without. For the Above is exalted by the Below." The last phrase is of special importance, for it reminds you that we humans easily slip into preferential judgments. We may assume the Above is better than the Below.

Above and Below, Without and Within, are not opposites. They are dynamic reflections that interact in the creative process we call the Universe. If you judge Above as being better than Below, the wisdom of the teaching gets lost.

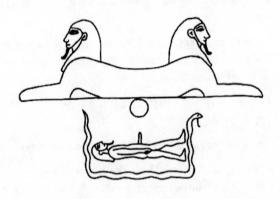

The Source is Oneness

Behind all apparent duality is that deeper Oneness that is the Source of All Things. Your phallus charged by Male Erotic Alchemy gives you the actual, direct experience of this singular reality. Indeed, all forms such as your body arise, change, and eventually dissolve back into the nothingness from which they arise—a no-thingness rich with limitless possibilities that await the opportunity for expression...

Beliefs in afterlife or pre-life existence are personal choices. More important is to believe in this Life and in yourself. Among the most crucial bits of ancient, even prehistoric wisdom is the awareness that your penis connects you with the fact that everything is alive and everything is sacred!

Every erection of your penis is the resurrection of your whole body.
In a real sense Life is all that exists.
Life happens now.

Chapter Eight:

The Son and Father of All Things

"The Son and Father of All Things" describes your relationship of intimate and familial connection with everything in existence.

You and the Universe are both co-creative and self-creating at once.

This is the essence of alchemical teachings, and the most powerful secret is that by means of your phallus, you create the world and the world creates you. You are the alchemist, and your body is the crucible in which this amazing process takes place.

This is not about changing you into something you are not, rather it is the return to your essential self, the core of who you have always been, without false additions. The Holy Child within you lives in unashamed Original Innocence.

From the viewpoint of Male Erotic Alchemy you are perfect exactly as you are, and so is everyone else. You are perfect and yet you can make yourself even more wonderful! Do not seek to fix or change yourself. Allow the intense, sustained, high quality ecstasy itself to do the work. The major benefits come about naturally as byproducts of the process of self-pleasure as self-love.

This is the most important pursuit for men of Planet Earth at this time. Now is the time for you to practice these processes as your way of life.

The term "alchemy" in English derives through the Arabic *al-kimiya* from the ancient Egyptian *Khem Amsu*, which is another name for Menu (or Min), the primary and original phallic god of Egypt. Khem Amsu refers to the fertile black soil whose name became the ancient Egyptian term for their own country, *Kemi*, which means "black land" or "black soil."

Remember the story of Atum, Lord of the Primordial Mound? His mound is of this rich, incredibly fertile black soil from the heart of Africa!

Atum masturbates and ejaculates directly into his own mouth, then he emits the first duality of Creation. This corresponds energetically with the act of auto-fellatio that some men are actually capable of. You should not necessarily try to do this. It's only possible with relative ease for a small fraction of especially flexible men, about two or three men in a thousand. Of course, in the yogic "plow position" any man can ejaculate into his own mouth, even if he cannot suck his own penis. At any rate, this circular flow of erogenous feedback corresponds with Ouroboros, the ultimate image of self-reference and self-creation, which is essentially masturbatory.

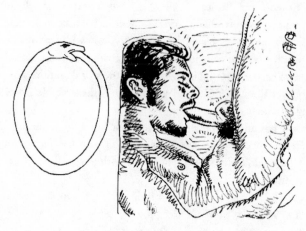

The Ouroboros energy and Lord Atum's beautiful Auto-fellatio

The Ouroboros, or Serpent that bites (or swallows) his own tail, rotates the cycle of self-aware and self-sustaining processes of Nature.

In Nature itself there is no good or evil, only the infinitely complex dance of energies. When imbalance occurs, natural forces converge to restore balance. This happens naturally and inevitably. Despite human attempts to control the outcome of events, deeper currents create reality.

Truth is not what we think it is. Truth is that rare bird that nests in the Tree of Life. It's the winged thing that the Serpent of Wisdom becomes when it climbs into the canopy where the simultaneous flowering and fruiting of Life occurs all the time.

The Serpent on the bough turns upon itself, and becomes the nest for its own egg; then the Dove hatches from the cloudy shell. The subtlety of the

Serpent becomes the wisdom of the Dove. Merged, they form the energy of the Feathered Serpent, Quetzalcoatl, the Morning Star, the Light Bringer, and Prince of the Breeze.

> Your own body IS the Tree of Life; your phallus IS the One Tree.
> Life-force energy and wisdom is the ascending Serpent Power.
> The thousand-petalled lotus crown opens atop your head.
> You feel deep peace that surpasses understanding.
> It rises from your deepest roots…
> Climbs the phallic axis…
> To the Blue Pearl…
> The Eye…
> "I"…

What IS Real Magick?

Real Magick can best be defined as "The art of altering consciousness at will."

As such, there's absolutely nothing supernatural or paranormal about Real Magick. Its power to bring about change in accord with your will stems from your alignment with the ways the natural world operates. Male Erotic Alchemy resembles ancient shamanic and tribal practices that open the individual to a direct experience of the powerful and profound mysteries of existence.

Male Erotic Alchemy employs Mindful Masturbation and semen retention to induce high erotic trance states to expand your consciousness, and allows you to create the realities you wish to experience.

Your pineal gland in the middle of your brain is activated in a manner that some traditions call the opening of the Third Eye, considered an organ of clairvoyance. The term "clairvoyant" literally means "to see clearly," and as such is not a paranormal faculty. Clarity is really the key to everything you want in your life.

As a Male Erotic Alchemist you employ Real Magick; in this way you are empowered to transform yourself and the reality you inhabit.

Connect Earth and Sky in Your Body

Because you are a human male, your body, your phallus, the core of your manifest energy aligns itself naturally with the vertical, rising energy that moves from the minus (–) pole of Below toward the plus (+) pole Above.

Keep in mind: these qualities of direction and charge have nothing to do with preferences such as undesirable or desirable, bad or good. They are more in the order of electrical charges. The direction is in relation to gravitation on the planet's surface.

Metaphysical teachings often fall into the same trap as religious teachings, by favoring one or the other of this dynamic duality. For example, darkness may be assigned negative qualities, while light is positive. Positive (+) and negative (–) are simply integral, dynamic, inter-creative aspects of the whole.

Likewise the social partnership with both women and men is necessary in human groups for overall balance.

Human females have a particular strength that human males often lack. Women naturally create a kind of Sisterhood. Even among women with no direct blood relation, deep bonds of friendship form and emotional intimacy is shared. When a woman faces a trauma or terrible loss, her "Sister" will do whatever she can to provide support, even shelter and company.

Men can learn from such Sisterhoos about how to create true Brotherhood: a genuine, sincere, and effective mutual support system. Partly due to cultural conditioning about the nature of "masculinity" and homophobia, when a buddy faces a trauma or terrible loss, his bud may express intense sympathy at first, yet often only briefly before he flees.

He feels too awkward with the emotions to stay the course.

The most effective way to begin to dissolve emotional damage due to traumatic personal history and acquired erroneous beliefs about the nature of "masculinity" is to simply surrender to the flow of erotic ecstasy through your male body.

Drop all resistance to that charge of irresistible, limitless bliss that pure penile pleasure generates. This energy circulates root-to-crown, out the top of your head, down around your outside as a torus or donut-shape, like magnetic field-lines. The ongoing flow envelopes you from head-to-toes, then curves back inward below your feet to re-circulate upward through your body again.

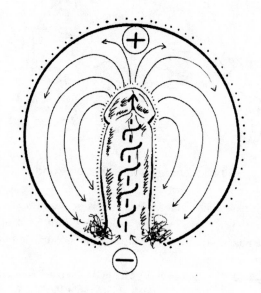

The Phallocentric Universe

During this kind of pure penile pleasure you enter a totally phallocentric Universe. The energy that flows through and around your erection becomes all that exists. When you stand upright in full arousal, your spine parallels this axis of rising male energy. When you lie flat on your back and aroused, as in the Yogic Corpse Pose or the Osiris Bed vignettes your erection parallels the same World Axis.

The perfect mythic image for this process is painted clearly in your mind's eye with the account earlier in this book of the Heliopolitan Creation story. Atum stands and masturbates as the ongoing process of Creation. His grandson Geb, the Lord of Earth, reclines on the ground with his fully erect penis aimed vertically at the zenith above where his sister Nut, the Lady of Sky, wears her twinkling, gemmed form as Nuit, the Lady of the Stars.

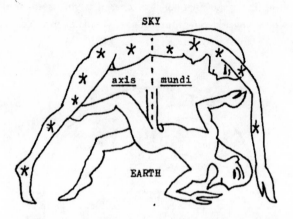

The Phallic Energy connects Earth and Sky

The Egyptians considered the erect penis or phallus to be a spiritual umbilical cord that connects every male body with its cosmic Source. Consider the blissful sensations provided by this spiritual umbilical as your universal sustenance.

The Starseed that conceives all Life and originates forms comes into existence from non-existence through the Cosmic Phallus. From there the Starseed emerges into the Cosmic Womb of space and time and thus the Universe is born.

In this sense, you *are* the Universe.

The Threefold Phallic Energy

Here is another way to understand how Male Erotic Alchemy amplifies your phallic energy. The flow of charged energy from − to + operates at every imaginable level, from subatomic spin-states, to revolving planets, stars and galaxies, to the universal whole.

In your body the − to + energy flow operates on these three levels: **1.)** Your erect penis itself, is charged with ecstasy, from the root within your perineum to the crown of the glans. **2.)** During penile arousal your spinal column and brain (the entire central nervous system) also enacts such a − to

+ flow, with signals that travel both ways up and down along your spine. **3.)** Your entire body when you stand upright to stimulate your phallus merges your energy field with the World Axis; you become the Rainbow Bridge that connects Earth with Sky in a full spectrum of chakras.

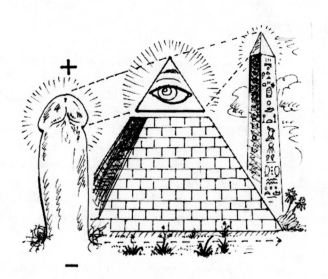

Penis, Pyramid and Obelisk

In Egypt the form of the pyramid crowns the tall slender obelisk, which is the Phallus of Lord Geb. In this connection you can recognize the true inner significance of the Eye in the Triangle atop the pyramid. It is your most intense connection with the Divine that levitates your matter above all mundane concerns and suffering. It is the special sensitivity of your glans penis, which also sends bliss through all of those levels.

One in Three; Three in One.

The Three corresponding "levels" of the − to + flow of phallic energy are actually One. They reinforce one another. The ecstatic feedback of this threefold phallic energy constructively increases the bliss within your entire body…

The doors of perception are cleansed and you see things as they are: *infinite!*

Alchemical Transformation through Mindful Masturbation

The practice of Mindful Masturbation becomes Male Erotic Alchemy when you begin to utilize the incredibly high erotic states and more advanced skills such as semen retention, to bring about lasting changes within you and without you. Your erotic energy empowers Male Solosex Magick, or partnered Sex Magick.

The aim of Male Erotic Alchemy is to perform a kind of depth psychology therapy upon yourself. Depth psychology is powerful and profound because it explores the relationship between the conscious and unconscious mind, and it also honors mythic archetypes. However Male Erotic Alchemy does not operate through traditional talk therapy or psychoanalysis... rather, it integrates your parts naturally during the total surrender to high erotic states.

As nervous system signals circulate, mental and emotional and physical energy is unblocked and released from those forms of insecurity and lack of self-love that prevent your further growth; then the ecstasy itself does the Great Work of alchemical transformation for you.

How do you get there?

Male Erotic Alchemy includes Mindful Masturbation and Male Solosex Magick to deliberately minimize the thought-processes of the mental sphere, to interrupt the incessant mental chatter, the story telling of ongoing inner dialogue. Over time your bliss simply dissolves much of that extraneous thinking, and the false identity it frequently reinforces.

Sufficient high-quality bliss clears the slate and cleans the brain.

Over time your focus becomes overwhelmingly constructive, self-empowering, and life enhancing. You no longer feed energy to negativity or poor self-esteem. From this new, healthier perspective you regenerate in a renewed form.

Neurotic habits, dysfunctional patterns of low self-esteem, rampant egotism and other less desirable traits simply shrivel up and dissipate from neglect.

Ordinarily you keep dysfunctional patterns of behavior in place by feeding them mental, emotional and physical energy. Everyone human does this—in no way are you unique or flawed in this manner. This is the human condition, a launch pad for all conscious evolution.

It is no accident or coincidence that you are reading this now, and yet this is not about intellectual understanding, rather it concerns the actual experience this inspires.

With this process of Male Erotic Alchemy, the nature of your limited "self" as an ego construct becomes crystal clear. Your personality can be seen as the creation of numerous opinions, attitudes and identification with various forms, such as appearance, job, possessions, accomplishments, or roles. They are all temporary.

There is nothing wrong with any of the elements of your ego, except that awareness helps you recognize they are not who and what you are. Your ego is not your enemy, rather it's an aspect of your human self that you may not want to have in control of your reactions. Better to befriend your ego, and make it an ally.

This allows your focus to return to your authentic, essential being: who and what you really are.

How to Deal with Guilt and Shame

Clear logic tells you that you have no good reason to feel any kind of guilt or shame about your body, your sexuality, and your penis. However, you may still feel some inhibitions or inabilities to fully celebrate yourself without any reservations. If so, this is due to a mix of conditioning and possibly even brain imprints.

If such limiting factors as guilt and shame persist, it is because you *feel* them, and this is not your fault. Feeling feeds a lot of energy into such patterns as poor self-esteem, uncertainty, and fear, and keeps them in place or even strengthens them. Logic, reason, psychoanalysis cannot really do much to help with this.

A truly effective approach for dealing with these feelings is to make the choice to treat yourself extremely well. Turn your attention from such doubts and fears to creating and generating extremely good feelings within yourself.

Masturbate mindfully without ejaculating often, so you keep the charge. This will eventually burn away and replace your guilt and shame with good feelings about your body, your sexuality, and your penis.

When you can say, "I AM that I AM becoming," in full awareness of your own divinity, you can actually experience your erection as the universal axis, the flow between – and + on all levels.

Even the scientific description of the expanding Universe insists that the center of the Universe is everywhere; it is always where you are. This is the truth no matter who you are or where you are. You are the center of the Universe; no more so or less so than anyone or anything else. The center is everywhere. With this realization you experience a marvelous liberation from separation and limitation!

Everything you experience as being "out there" happens within you.
Without you and within you in relation to your body are truly One.
One in Three; Three in One can be stated: 1 = 3; 3 = 1.
Without and within merely reflect one another.
There is no "out there" there.
Yet you exist—for now.
You are...
...the Universe!

All of Alchemy in One Yantra: Dr. Dee's Monad

Dr. John Dee, his son Arthur, and Arthur's friend Sir Thomas Browne of the 16th and 17th centuries were pioneers of Western Sex Magick (among other things) who laid the groundwork for the Male Erotic Alchemy you can practice now in the 21st Century!

Queen Elizabeth I of England presided over her times as something of a living goddess. The Italian Renaissance had recently unleashed monumental shifts of Western culture toward both its classical roots and the foundations for today's scientific paradigm. Elizabeth Tudor was also called "The Virgin Queen, Gloriana, and Good Queen Bess"—as a sort of Triple Goddess of her aspects.

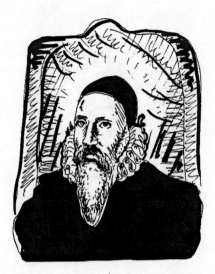

Dr. John Dee

One amazing man of this era was Dr. John Dee. Officially a "consultant" or "advisor" to the Queen on matters of science, he also served as her royal astrologer. This was the case at a time when witchcraft, traffic with spirits, and the practice of Magick were officially illegal. Dee was a true Renaissance man: mathematician, astronomer, geographer, navigator, book collector, philosopher, plus he was credited with originating the concept of Britain as an imperial power.

He was also an alchemist.

Dee lived from 1527-1608 or 1609. The uncertain year of the great man's demise while he lived in Manchester indicates the obscurity into which he had fallen by that time, after a long period of fame, acclaim and notoriety. A remarkable man of great learning and a vast scope of interests, Dee straddled both science and Magick at a time when the two realms of study were only beginning to diverge.

He collected the greatest library in England of his day, indeed, among the most extensive in all of Europe. His collection attracted the interest of many scholars who often visited him. Dee's library became a center of learning outside of the official universities. When Elizabeth was crowned in 1558, Dee had already become an advisor and tutor to her. His star ascended with hers, and he influenced the great voyages of discovery then happening.

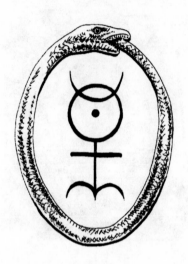

Dee's Monad in the Phallic Brotherhood Logo

In 1564 Dee published *Monas Hieroglyphica*, a text in Latin—which was the lingua franca of the day—as an explanation of a mystical glyph that he had designed or derived from his own visions. The glyph condenses all the cosmic symbols of the planets, the zodiac, and the elements into a single image. "Dee's Monad," as the sign came to be known, expresses the mystical Oneness of Creation. It serves as a sort of embryonic symbol from which all sorts of esoteric and astrological signs can be derived.

Some say that the deeper and higher significance of Dee's Monad is unknown because the living oral and initiatory traditions of its meanings were lost. *And yet it can speak for itself!* With a basic grasp of Sacred Number and the archetypal energies inherent in signs and shapes, the deeper and higher significance of Dee's Monad can be recovered. The Monad acts as a revelatory conduit of universal truth.

This remarkable sign sums up all of Alchemy within a single *Yantra*.

Yantra is the Sanskrit word for "instrument," "machine," or "device," and it refers to any image or form that has structure or organization, generally used to balance or focus the mind. For example, a Tibetan Mandala, or sacred image that usually involves both circular and square forms of geometry can be called a Yantra. Both control and liberation emanate from any given Yantra. In fact, the body itself is said to be a Yantra.

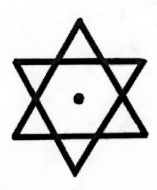

The Great Device of Tantra

The Maha Yantra (The Great Device) of Tantric tradition is the intersection of upward and downward pointing triangles with a point at their common center. This unification of the Below with the Above indicates the union of the Mountain God or Shiva (consciousness) with The Great Divine Mother (energy) as the ongoing process of their bliss that forms the central dynamo of Creation.

This is the non-duality of Oneness.

Though some Tantric teachers and practitioners consider this Maha Yantra to be a specific symbol of heterosexual intercourse performed as a Magick rite, its deeper and higher significance indicates that duality merges back into Oneness.

Like the Maha Yantra, Dee's Monad has precisely six lines and a dot. Similarly, the Monad is the living image of the universal design, the "formative blueprint" so-to-speak, of the cosmic order.

The Monad reflects the essential pattern of how energy flows in the Universe.

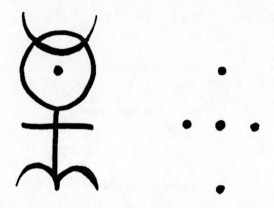

The Monad is the Essential Pattern of All Things

Look at it and you see: the central axis that rises from Below, emerges from between the two semi-circular crescents, like the stalk of a growing plant that stands between two emerging leaves. Hidden in this Monad are the five points of the quincunx that will soon reappear as the story unfolds below.

The axis lifts to meet the horizontal crossbar at the crossroads where you stand, the place between worlds, the place where the phallic god stands, upright, centered, balanced upon the downward pull of gravity.

The axis continues upward and meets the solar circle with a central point. This symbol by itself is also called the "circumpunct," a dot centered in a circle that represents unity or Oneness, as well as the Sun, and a simple model of an atom.

However this solar circle is crowned by an intersecting crescent that rests atop its radiance and aims its lunar horns above. This overlap of circle and semi-circle enacts the eclipse, that integral connection between solar and lunar aspects of the cosmic wheels in whose turnings our existence is ordained.

In essence, consider the Monad as a diagram of Shiva: *his crossed legs are the twin arches Below, his spine rises to his arms, and atop his solar head is perched the lunar crescent.*

The central axis of phallic energy connects Below with Above, plus the reverse, and also connects Within with Without. The axis of energy rises from the root of the planetary core through your body to connect with your head where you also connect with the universal.

Dr. Dee described the basic significance of the Monad as combining the solar and lunar signs with the four elements in the form of the cross. However the Monad has far greater subtlety for those not deflected by his casual simplification.

In reality the Monad contains aspects of all sorts of signs, in condensed and overlaid potency. It acts as a sort of cosmic sperm cell for the Male Erotic Alchemist alert to its endless nuances.

A most effective means to expand your awareness of the Monad's power is to masturbate mindfully while you gaze upon it. Even more powerful, once you know its basic figure well, simply visualize it, and hold it in your mind's eye while you practice Mindful Masturbation.

Dee enclosed the Monad within an oval to suggest the egg of the living Universe.

For the Male Erotic Alchemist, you find its universal potency perfected by enclosure within the Ouroboros, the Serpent that bites his own tail, the Complete One: self-creative, self-sustaining, self-regenerative.

Arthur Dee and Sir Thomas Browne

Dr. Dee understood and practiced a European version of what we now call Sex Magick that reached the savants of the Western World through secretive means of transmission because the dominant religions of the day frowned upon such practices. Some elements of this alchemical Sex Magick traveled into Europe when the Moorish culture entered Spain. During the Crusades, The Knights Templar, the Cathars and Troubadours helped to transmit these traditions westward from the Far East.

This Western Sex Magick included elements found in East Indian Tantra and Chinese Taoist Sexual Cultivation, such as using the breath as a tool for conscious engineering, and the practice of semen retention, which allows you to absorb the erotic energy generated during penile stimulation.

These practices had to be kept closely guarded secrets in Elizabethan times, despite the burgeoning "scientific" attitudes that emerged from the late Renaissance. The Inquisition that also grew partly out of the Crusades continued to demonize anything other than its own doctrines and dogmas.

The Protestant churches that had broken away from the Mother Church of Rome proved no more tolerant of such mystical and alchemical teachings.

Thus John Dee could only pass on the deepest and highest aspects of the Hieroglyphic Monad through an extremely secretive oral tradition and an experiential initiation into the Male Mysteries of the Phallus. In metaphorical, yet explicit terms he describes the circulation of the erotic energy within the body in Theorem XVIII of his treatise *The Hieroglyphic Monad*. Yet only the awareness that his subject was actually what we now call Male Erotic Alchemy makes this clear.

Dee used the process of Sex Magick to energize himself and to refine his conscious awareness to uncommon depths and heights. Still he never achieved quite the kind of "psychic attunement" he aspired to in order to delve even deeper and higher into the mysteries of the cosmos. He sought mediums and what we would now call channels or psychics to help. Still, he obtained no dramatic results until he hooked up with a character he knew as Edward Kelley.

With the help of Kelley to do the crystal gazing, Dee produced dramatic results, with "Enochian" or Angelic Magick, which involved elaborate ritual practices to alter consciousness and to contact beings considered "angels" or "spirits." This they did with dramatic effect at a time when it was technically illegal. Many witnesses also became convinced that these two men actually transformed common metals into precious metals. The results of this team proved so striking that their work formed much of the basis for modern ritual magic, including the works of Aleister Crowley and the Golden Dawn.

One startling thing about the "Enochian" or "Angelic" Magick these men recorded is that it simply works. It's the real deal.

With Kelley, Dee traveled to the European mainland where he became involved with several rulers who sought his services. The two men evidently performed alchemical transmutations. They changed pewter vessels into silver good enough for the Jewish goldsmiths to purchase the metal. However, Kelley had a shady past and dubious morals.

Eventually he persuaded Dee that they were supposed to swap wives on the orders of a higher power, and soon after that, Dee broke with him.

Dee returned to England, while Kelley apparently died during an attempt to escape from prison.

The good doctor tried to continue his communication with the spirits using the help of his son Arthur, then eight or nine years of age. Though Dee felt the boy had special gifts and anointed him as Kelley's successor, the boy could not see or hear anything through the crystals.

Regardless of that, Arthur grew up as a protégé of his father. He became a scholarly student of the alchemical arts, and his father initiated him into the mysteries of the Hieroglyphic Monad. Arthur became a physician as his public career, though his credentials were often questioned. Still he enjoyed great success. For some years he lived in Russia, as an advisor to the Tsar.

Like his father, Arthur practiced the Sex Magick in which he did not ejaculate except to conceive yet another of his many children. He experienced life as "The Son and Father of All Things," which is the energy state induced by semen retention that brings about an ongoing sense of relationship with everything in existence.

Years after his father's death, when Arthur returned to England, he settled near a friend named Sir Thomas Browne. Arthur had produced a scholarly collection of works on alchemy, a subject of great interest to Browne.

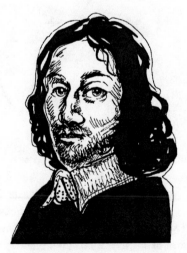

Sir Thomas Browne

Arthur also passed on his initiation into the mysteries of the Hieroglyphic Monad to Browne, who likewise evidently practiced the Sex Magick of semen retention to refine conscious awareness. Browne later wrote a treatise called *The Garden of Cyrus*. This famous piece of magnificent prose describes the author's direct perception of the weave of energies in Nature that his aroused and elevated awareness revealed to him. That energetic weave is the "loom" or "warp" of the Sanskrit root for the term "Tantra."

Browne describes the realization that the world we live in is actually Paradise, the Garden of Eden, if we have eyes to see and ears to hear. We never left the Garden except in our minds as we developed complex language and dualistic concepts that seem to separate us from Nature.

This great man described his own experience of the return to Paradise that occurs when the arbitrary boundaries of belief between human nature and Nature itself dissolve as the human male cultivates vital energy in his body in order to recover his Original Innocence.

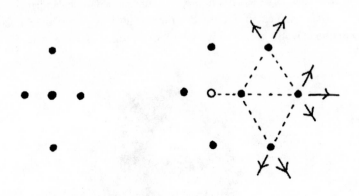

The Quincunx and the Energetic Weave of Tantric Nadis

The Garden of Cyrus elaborates Browne's direct experience inspired by his initiation into the mysteries of the Hieroglyphic Monad. He demonstrates that from the quincunx of five points the sacred geometry of Life radiates throughout the world of manifestation. Living energy weaves through all forms of living things in energetic filaments called "nadis" in Tantrick terms. Browne shows how this geometry extends into "diamond" and "parallelogram" patterns that pervade plant life and growth, and indeed throughout Nature from crystal lattices of minerals, to animal forms.

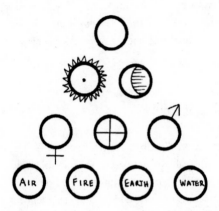

Sacred Number and Creation (The Tetractys)

The triangles, diamonds and parallelograms weave both Sacred Number and sacred geometry all through the world you live in. No aspect has a fixed or absolute meaning. All are fluid and flow through variations of where they appear and how they interact. The only constant of such imagery is the vertical phallic energy that connects Below with Above.

The Garden of Cyrus written by Sir Thomas Brown preserves in its own terms the "long-lost" oral and experiential initiation of the Hieroglyphic Monad: the Male Mysteries of the Phallus. This unlocked for Browne the alchemical life of living as "The Son and Father of All Things," in direct relations to everything.

Due to their context, both of the Dees, father and son, and Browne had to write of these matters in code. Yet their writings and the events of their lives make it plain that among western Europeans, they pioneered what we now call the Secret of the Golden Phallus. These three men knew of the Male Mysteries and practiced a form of Western Sex Magick. The stories of their lives, their marriages, their connections with one another, along with their characteristic energy, wisdom, magickal potency and human intensity all tend to confirm this as well.

Though they were married men and considered themselves Christians, both of the Dees, Kelley, and Browne enjoyed abundant sexual activity and yet they must have seldom ejaculated, and practiced semen retention to alter their consciousness. A careful reading of John Dee's treatise *The Hieroglyphic Monad* and Arthur Dee's *Fasciculus Chemicus* and Browne's *The Garden of Cyrus* confirms that these men knew and practiced this secret.

Seek the Root of "I"

Where do you fit into the bigger picture of the Universe? For one thing, you are an animal. You are part of the natural world. And within this, you emerged along with your remarkably evolved penis!

Among the most astonishing tales of modern science is the emergence of five or six major kingdoms of life—not only the plant and animal kingdoms, but also three or four more! These kingdoms remain debatable in terms of extent and number.

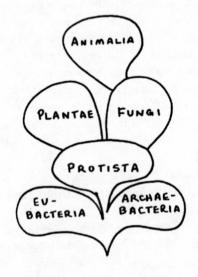

Ancestral Tree of Biology

This kind of diagram offers only a provisional image of the relationships between what we call kingdoms, while in fact the whole of Life is One. Still, like the digits of your own hand, or members of your immediate family and household, its form facilitates function. One notable aspect of this particular family tree of Life is the emergence of the Animal Kingdom not from Plants, but from Fungi.

The earliest ancestors of what we now call animals may have been fungi that developed an ability to surround their food with a membrane in order to absorb nutrients, the beginnings of a digestive process.

In fact, the story goes back all the way to what some consider the beginning...

This Universe apparently emerged in the event that we call the Big Bang some *13.7 billion years ago.*

Stardust has evolved over inconceivably long, yet apparently finite expanses of time. From that beginning about nine billion years passed until the formation of the Earth within an immense, whirling disc of plasma at whose center the star we now call the Sun coalesced as the hub. Then, less than a billion years after the molten, virgin planet congealed its orb from the plasma, something triggered the emergence of Life. The timeline of evolutionary emergence from the first living cells to you and your remarkable penis shows a dramatic acceleration...

3.5 billion years ago the first living cells emerged. The earliest amino acids, and precursors of DNA such as RNA eventually spun proteins into membranes and began the fabrication of fantastic cellular architecture in the form of the earliest plants, which resembled today's blue green algae.

2 to 1.5 billion years ago sexual reproduction began with yeast-like organisms. Cyanobacteria began to form long green strands and built civilizations in the form of bumpy green mounds called stromatolites. They used photosynthesis to weave sunlight and available elements into sugars and proteins.

A byproduct of this process was oxygen and the early cyanobacteria became so successful and generated so much oxygen that the young planet was actually in danger of rusting away and as it grew toxic to itself.

So the genetic wisdom of DNA extruded from the biomass, the first single-celled creatures we would call animals that could absorb and metabolize oxygen.

550 million years ago with the first multi-celled creatures the formation of basic body structure arose, sac-like forms that resembled jellyfish.

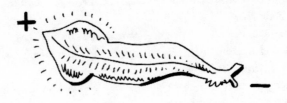

A prehistoric worm called "Pikea"

530 million years ago with worm-like creatures, the definition of a head-end (+) that contained a primitive brain and a tailend (–) with a lengthwise central nerve cord that connected the ends emerged. The worm-like creatures had a mouth at one end, a simple digestive tract, and expelled waste through the anus at the other end.

480 million years ago fish developed movable jaws, eyes and gills, fins and a tail that provided effective feeding and mobility.

375 million years ago the basic form of fish-like creatures already contained all the essential parts of a human body as they emerged from aquatic living partly on land, with their fins deployed like simple legs.

359 million years ago the first true amphibians appear.

310 million years ago reptilian forms emerged from amphibians.

210 million years ago warm-blooded mammalian ancestors arose, that gave live birth to their dependent young and cared for them until they matured.

60 million years ago early primate ancestors scampered through treetops of the Ancestral Forest Primeval, in this case an actual place in sub-Saharan Africa. These tiny squirrelly creatures developed binocular vision as their eyes moved to the fronts of their faces. Their tiny feet developed rudimentary thumbs to provide an effective grip.

20 million years ago monkeys that retained tails for balance in trees, and the apes that lost their tails as they developed greater agility on the ground, and part-time upright mobility, diverged.

10 million years ago gorillas diverged from a common ancestor of the other great apes, including us.

8 million years ago the bonobos (our closest living relatives) branched off from the chimpanzees and also from us. We resemble the bonobos in that we are sexually active all the time, rather than going into periods of heat, as chimpanzees do. We resemble both the somewhat aggressive and violent chimps, and the highly sexed, far more peaceful and nonviolent bonobos. Worthy of emulation by us in this way, the bonobos frequently release social tension and resolve conflicts by enjoying sexual pleasure instead of fighting. That's their attitude adjustment!

5 million years ago our regular bipedal locomotion and bigger-than-ever brains encouraged manipulation with opposable-thumbed hands, and the beginnings of symbolic spoken language.

1.5 million years ago human ancestors learned to use fire.

1.2 million years ago humans developed dark skin and had lost most body hair.

350,000 years ago the Neanderthal branch of humanity left Africa through the Middle East and generally migrated north and west into Europe.

200,000 years ago what we now consider modern humans, physically, had appeared in Africa.

60-50,000 years ago is probably about the time ancestral humans left Africa and bred with Neanderthals as they went. The major flow passed around the Arabian Sea into South India before they radiated from there.

40,000 years ago ancestors of modern humans entered Australia and Europe.

30-25,000 years ago the independent Neanderthals died out, though some of their genes survived in modern humans, especially Europeans.

12,000 years ago light skin evolved among humans, and when the "Hobbits" of Flores Island in Indonesia died out, that left us the only living species of our genus.

Now all humans on the planet, regardless of superficial variations in color and physical features are a single race and species, far more similar than we are different. All humans share more complex and intentional sexual activities than any of our animal kindred. The personal and social purposes of orgasm among human beings seem to reflect an evolutionary heritage that parallels our developing intelligence.

The complexity of our sexual behaviors and the quest for orgasmic reward that is not purely instinctive and reproductive must have also inspired the general development of self-awareness and intelligence at the same time. Simultaneously our intelligence evolved the complexity and diversity of our sexual expressions.

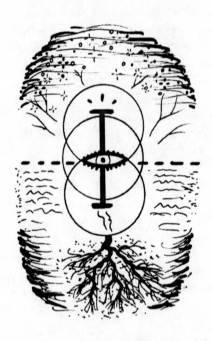

Seeking the Root of "I" (Three Worlds: Upper, Middle and Lower)

You like every other human being, are a unique and individual universe, the living heir and embodiment of the entire history not only of Life on Earth, but also of the Living Universe. "I" as used here means the Universal Self, rather than the personal and individual self of the personality, mind and body. As such, this I is the "I AM" or Creator, centered within what humans view as three worlds: Above, Middle, and Below; Heaven, Earth, Underworld. The same center is within you. A scientific version simply locates you on the planetary surface as the microcosm of the macrocosm, a being that reflects the same principles at work throughout the cosmos.

You embody the entire story of biological evolution from the first amino acids and single cells through your personal parentage. Your body of organs, cells, molecules, and atoms also retains the encoded memory of the whole story of the cosmos from what we call the Big Bang to *now*.

As fascinating and insightful as the timeline above may seem, it is still only a story, though based on recent evidence and reason. It must not be mistaken for the profound and powerful ancestral mysteries within you that it points toward. Those inner mysteries are your actual, undeniable truth.

Nature loves to repeat and recycle successful forms, and with this awareness the resemblance of your penis to the fruiting body of fungi that we call a "mushroom," takes on new meaning.

In fact, fungi mostly manifest as mycelium, far less obvious and far more important than the beautiful growth of mushrooms that we all know. Mycelium is single-celled and forms long thread-like weavings in the soil, particularly in association with trees and forests. An overturned rock or log may reveal some gauzy white floss of mycelium, which turns out to be crucial to the health of living soils.

An even more amazing aspect of mycelium is that it acts as a sort of nervous system or something like an organic Internet for natural environments worldwide. Mycelium connects and communicates vital information among living things of all the world's forests. The mushrooms that can appear so swiftly after rainfall are only temporary fruiting bodies. They may broadcast spores over the surface, though most of the fungus is actually the unseen mycelium beneath the surface.

Your body contains many parallels with aspects of Nature, including the mycelium and its mushrooms. The mycelium resembles your nervous system, mostly within your skin, and your penis resembles the fruiting body of the fungus, called a mushroom. Ponder this analogy with humorous detachment while you contemplate your beautiful penis and in a relaxed manner, masturbate and breathe deeply.

On the deepest and highest level you *are* your family tree!

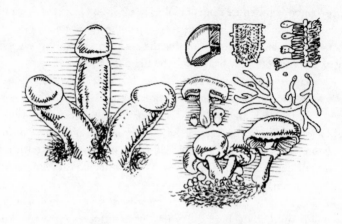

Nature Repeats Successful Forms

Your penis is the original sacred mushroom, the food of the gods. Just as some psychoactive fungi may have triggered the evolution of human consciousness, thought and feelings in the past, your penis now plays an important role in your conscious evolution as an individual.

All mythologies, all Ancestors, all possible forms are within you.
Verbal language cannot get you there or even show the way.
Your penis provides you with direct access now.
You are the Son and Father of All Things.
The truth is between your legs.

CHAPTER NINE:

CREATE THE WORLD

Creation did not happen 13.7 billion years ago, or a mere several thousand, rather it is happening now. Creation is always present, ongoing in the material atoms, stardust, molecules, cells, organs, and in the organic form of your human body.

Pure penile pleasure does a lot more for you than to feel incredibly, indescribably good. It transforms your experience of living from struggle, coping and managing, to profound enjoyment, gratitude, and grace. Grace means shameless and guilt-free—you need not validate your existence or earn forgiveness. Grace is simply yours.

Original Innocence is your default state. All you really need to do is work on loving yourself, get clarity from within, and the rest follows.

Erotic Re-Imprinting

Two basic processes strongly determine the kind of reality you experience: conditioning and imprinting. To understand the difference reveals what is possible through Male Erotic Alchemy.

Conditioning is actually no more than acquired beliefs that shape the kind of reality you experience. From birth your caretakers condition you, often with the best of intentions, to accept certain agreements about the way things work in your world. Some of these beliefs help you function in the world and among people, however you are also taught much that is merely common opinions. Some of what you learn is questionable or blatantly untrue.

Among common agreements and assumptions are that nobody is perfect, especially *you*. Boys are strong and tough, girls are weak and sensitive. (Or they *should* be!) You can't always get what you want. Life is difficult. You have to work hard for a living, even if you hate your work. You have to earn the love of others by your behavior. You are not attractive. You do not deserve love. You do not deserve abundance. You are born sinful.

All of those are opinions learned about your world and yourself, and about 99% of such beliefs have no validity at all!

Conditioning is merely ideas and beliefs, however this has powerful determining effects upon the quality of your life experience. At the same time, conditioning can change, just as your opinions can change. In reality, many people do not actually change much after their teenage years when certain opinions and behavior patterns tend to become fixed for life. With the onset of adulthood, many people stop growing and seldom change.

Yet conditioning, as limiting as it can be, is relatively easy to change compared with brain imprints. Though imprinting in humans remains somewhat speculative and controversial, based on the evidence presented below, I will speak of it as a reality. Here I also use the word "imprint" as a noun, though it is more often used as a verb.

The best-known example of imprinting among animals, perhaps, is that of ducklings hatched in the presence of a person instead of the parent duck. The ducklings imprint the person as their parent and follow that person around, wanting to be fed and cared for. This happens because the hatchling's brain and nervous system are so open and sensitized upon emergence from the shell that it arbitrarily imprints anything present larger than itself, as its parental figure.

We now have reasons to believe that our own experience as human beings is also strongly determined by imprints.

The imprint is like a complete picture of the quality of your experience at a key moment. It seems that your brain and nervous system takes a flash photo of your reality at that specific interval of imprint vulnerability. This can be a largely positive, somewhat neutral or largely negative world-view. It exists at the unconscious level, however it strongly influences how you view things in your conscious mind.

The imprint is a much deeper determinant of your reality than conditioning is, and more challenging to change. However when you understand this and realize that you can change your imprints through the process called re-imprinting, to simply know this begins to transform your reality far more profoundly than merely changing your opinions.

Our understanding of imprints and re-imprinting in human experience comes from several sources. To combine the information from those sources yields a compelling paradigm that empowers you to create your world for optimum function, enjoyment and success. The imprinting of animals first became well known from the work of the scientist Konrad Lorenz, who demonstrated the famous example of the hatchlings.

Later experiments with psychedelic psychotherapy led to theories that humans are also subject to imprinting, especially during the critical period of a psychedelic session. Dr. Timothy Leary, PhD proposed a model of multiple developmental imprints during a human lifetime. Leary maintained that the critical periods of imprinting came at birth, the toddler stage, while learning symbolic communication, and at puberty. He also suggested further potential imprints that remain latent in most people, and that may unfold with our future evolution.

Many human brain imprints seem to simply happen during the course of your life at key moments of vulnerability, caused by the process of growing up, or some kind of health crisis, or various forms of stress that can trigger re-imprinting. Imprinting and re-imprinting seem to happen when the body and brain are flooded with certain hormones and neurotransmitter chemicals. Those who know how to induce this deliberately can impose an imprint on a person using various techniques.

An imprint in itself may be good, indifferent, or bad in its effect. Thus, once you clearly understand the process it must be employed with loving care and careful deliberation. The same process of re-imprinting may be used to cure serious addictive behaviors, heal psychological abuse, or it can be *mis*used to brainwash vulnerable individuals into cultish belief-systems. In fact, the "boot-camp" of basic training employed by military organizations is an effective and dramatic form of re-imprinting.

The most useful insights into how imprinting works actually come from the early experiments of psychedelic drug therapy conducted during the 1950s and the early 1960s. At the time such substances remained legal in the USA and researchers developed extremely effective therapeutic practices.

In carefully arranged sessions, patients were informed of what to expect, prepared, and the sessions conducted in pleasant, safe surroundings with experienced guides, correct dosages of pure pharmaceutical psychedelics, and plenty of time for the process to unfold fruitfully. No distractions, such as telephones, or social obligations were allowed to intrude. The guides monitored the patient carefully, so that if the patient became upset or disoriented, their attention could be positively re-directed.

Though the actual session often proved intense and overwhelming to the patient, upon emergence from the psychedelic state the patient was encouraged to relax. They were urged to reflect and allow the experience to gradually integrate with the return to more normal states of consciousness.

Many who had suffered extremely serious problems before such a session, received substantial and lasting benefits, which continue to this day. In other words, in terms of effectiveness, the early experimental therapies proved extremely promising and successful! Unfortunately, the mainstream culture of the times was not ready for this. Soon the publicity became a frenzy of notoriety, careful experiments lapsed into a wild party, and eventually the psychedelic substances were legally banned.

Part of what had been learned was that reality as we experience it is an extremely complex and fragile construct of the mind—or more specifically of the state of your mind! Likewise, with the increasing militarism of the USA, the rise of certain religious cults, and several notorious kidnappings, the nature of brainwashing became clear. Brainwashing is merely a rather crude, yet effective form of re-imprinting.

The basics are simple. Social isolation and the removal of previous identity markers, combined with total dependence on caretakers, exhaustion, hunger and emotional stress leads to a kind of neurological flux, or imprint vulnerability. The military, religious cults, and some deviously canny kidnappers employ the same basic process. Isolate the individual from previous social contacts; remove familiar markers of identity and eliminate freedom of movement; keep inductees busy with exertion, sleeplessness, hunger and harassment.

Once the previous identity and basis for self-worth are dissolved, the caretakers or authorities find it easy to re-imprint the individual in a new belief system. "Privileges" and comforts are restored by increments and conditionally. A new role and identity of subservience to the belief system is created, and this becomes totally real for the individual. A person re-imprinted in this way is bonded to their authority figure like the duckling, and may obey without question. Illustrations of this are the notorious

Manson family brainwashings in the late 1960s and what happened to Patti Hearst after she was kidnapped in 1974.

Though re-imprinting can be put to such sinister uses, it also becomes tremendously empowering and beneficial when the same insights are put to constructive use in a life-enhancing manner for personal growth.

Re-imprinting tends to occur during times of stress, such as puberty, extreme illness or exhaustion, childbirth for a woman, or during a near death experience... and I have observed that re-imprinting can also take place during experiences of prolonged and intense erotic ecstasy.

Human development from birth to adulthood seems to involve a series of imprints that generally occur at the time of birth, during the crawling and toddling stage of infant development, while learning language and manipulative dexterity, and also a social-sexual imprint associated with the first major orgasmic experience of puberty.

Such developmental imprints are usually taken pretty much at random in today's cultures, though the rites of passage and shamanic rituals of many traditional societies often involve deliberately engineered re-imprinting.

Used wisely and lovingly, the process of re-imprinting can produce a more balanced, secure, confident individual, just as its misuse produces robotic and subservient behavior. In fact, the largely random manner in which most people take their imprints almost inevitably results in automated, somewhat dysfunctional behavior patterns.

Leary and his cohort Robert Anton Wilson described further imprints beyond the social-sexual one of physical maturity, such as a body awareness imprint, higher brain functions, the genetic wisdom of Nature, and even universal Oneness.

Most important for you, now, is the fact that you need no psychedelic drugs, no stress, no one to perform brainwashing, in order to re-imprint yourself for optimal function, health and happiness. You have everything you need to dissolve your old patterns of behavior and to open the doors of perception, with your male human body and the willingness to explore your erotic potential.

Male Erotic Alchemy can be employed to help you create the reality you wish to inhabit: Paradise, also known as Heaven on Earth, or the New Earth.

How to Train Your Penis

Just as the fingers of a musician learn increasing skills with ongoing practice and the playing of music, and the vocal cords of a singer are trained by singing, with the regular practice and exercise of Mindful Masturbation, you actually *train* your penis to give you ever-increasing quality and amounts of erotic ecstasy.

Yes, your penis learns!

The common jokes about "Men think with their penis," or "My penis has a mind of its own," actually contain some truth. Of course, your penis does not contain a full-fledged brain; still its head is richly endowed with exquisitely sensitive pleasure-receptor nerves, and through Penis Reflexology it does correspond with the head atop your shoulders. In that sense the glans is the "brain" of your penis.

So two heads are better than one! Your cranial brain can easily lead you into confusion and suffering, while the complex of nerves housed in the surface of your glans penis has the capacity to bring you back into balance, back into your center. The idea that a man's penis "misleads" him is the opposite of the truth! If you allow your sexual desire to cause you problems, this is your responsibility, and your penis cannot be blamed.

The quality of your pure penile pleasure can literally continue to increase and grow ever more refined—indefinitely. Consider what is called "neuroplasticity," in relation to your experience of pure penile pleasure. Until quite recently it was believed that nerves never regenerate and the brain cannot heal. Indeed after a certain age you do continue to lose brain cells progressively over time.

However, with an active mind and constant learning, your brain and nervous system continues to complexify, for the connections between the neurons, the fibers called axons and dendrites, continue to grow.

Neuroplasticity describes how new neural pathways are physically wired-into your brain when you are trained in a new behavior pattern.

What was considered irreparable damage in the past has been seen to be "wired around" or circumvented by new pathways with persistent practice and therapeutic exercise. Plus, in the treatment of obsessive-compulsive disorders the application of mindfulness proves far more humane and effective than aversion therapies of the past.

The study of behavioral re-training that employs mindfulness has produced measurable new neural pathways, which physically confirms the reality of neuroplasticity. Advanced brain imaging techniques evocatively called PET, fMRI and MEG have confirmed that new pathways are reinforced and strengthened in the brain.

Clearly when you begin to masturbate mindfully, which starts with paying full attention, noticing your habitual patterns and deliberately breaking them to explore new practices, you are also likely to generate new pathways in the nerves of your penis, its connection with the erectile center in your lower spine, and throughout your body and brain as you deliberately involve your entire body and mind as an erogenous zone.

My personal experience tends to confirm this, as I continue to discover new levels of ecstasy over the years. In this way, by your devotion to pure penile pleasure, you may also continually increase the capacity of your penis to provide ecstatic sensations.

To train your penis in this manner is its own reward. Until you begin to experience the ever-increasing refinements and intensity you are capable of, this may sound far-fetched.

Ask your penis about this—it knows better than your mind.

Intelligence Increase Between Your Legs

Your penis is not to be judged upon whether or not it literally has a brain, for it does not, however it embodies an important aspect of your overall intelligence. Your penis should not be judged at all, except as sacred!

By the concerted creation of high quality erotic ecstasy combined with cerebral intelligence, you begin to strengthen the capacity of your heart for feeling. The location of your heart lies literally in between your genitalia and your brain along the spinal column. This means that as you increase the two-way traffic of sensory-erotic signals that pass along your spine, your heart begins to bloom like the bud of a lotus flower that rises to the surface of murky waters and opens its inner fragrance to the light.

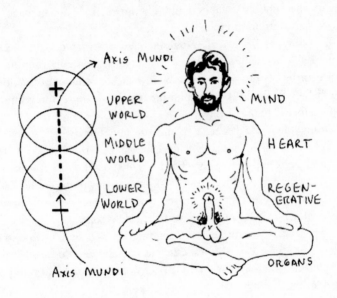

The Male Human Body and the Three Worlds

Here you see the gentle, effortless merging of all aspects of the Triple God; the triune view of the world, as having a Below, a Middle, and an Above; energy flows and flowers naturally and effortlessly from the minus (–) pole below to the plus (+) pole above and between them. Your body and your penis are radiant, luminous with life and divinity. In most tribal and shamanic traditions there are these same three worlds, Lower, Middle and Upper, or Underworld, Earth and Sky, that correspond with genitals, heart and mind, or with Moon, Sun and Stars.

Notice that all of these images come directly from actual, material and natural experience of the world you live in and from your body itself. This is the animal processing of your nervous system and metabolic energy and by the vegetative intelligence that operates on the surface of the planet within the biosphere.

To align your embodiment with this flow and growth and flowering is to enter the infinite dance of divine play.

Dreaming on the Cosmic Serpent

Among the most compelling images with roots deep and branches high in that marvelous Indus Valley culture is the image of Vishnu the Lord Sustainer as he reclines on the body of the Cosmic Serpent that swims in the Cosmic Ocean of Milk. This Serpent with multiple heads is essentially the Serpent Power or living energy and wisdom of the Universe itself as a material realm.

Vishnu's name means "The All-Pervading One," for all of the major avatars of much later Hindu and Buddhist tradition are said to be incarnations of him. His nature is omnipresent and liberating. Vishnu is the color of a rain-filled cloud, and he most often has four arms holding a lotus, mace, conch, and *chakra* or wheel. He also has an awesome Universal Form that is beyond the limits of ordinary human perception.

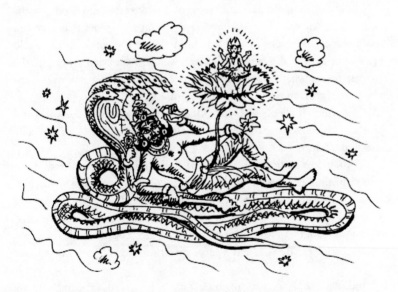

The Sustainer Reclines on the Cosmic Serpent

Vishnu reclines at ease upon the many-headed Cosmic Serpent, and from his body, at periodic intervals a lotus stalk extends to form a bud. The description and depiction sometimes indicates that the lotus emerges from the navel of Vishnu, only that is a later, prudish revision. It is actually the stalk of his phallus, and more accurately it emerges from between his legs.

Just as the Egyptian phallic god sometimes has an erection that is shown to emerge from his navel—in both cases the true significance is that of the phallus as a spiritual umbilical cord that connects the male body with its universal Source.

The lotus bud that extends from Vishnu's body grows to maturity and when the flower opens, upon its petals Lord Brahma is born. The Creator Brahma, with four faces and four arms, sits upright, and unlike most other Hindu gods, he holds no weapons. As he opens his eight eyes, the Universe comes into being. When he closes his eyes again, he sinks back into the flower, the bud closes and retreats back into the body of Vishnu.

This also parallels the Egyptian story of the birth of the Sun God, Ra, born from the heart of the Blue Lotus, Nefertum, which grows along the Nile River lagoons.

These stories signify the emergence of divinity from the depths of the unknown darkness, the void—or simply the unseen roots that give rise within matter and energy to a divine form, whose perception of the world is in itself creative. In quantum physics, a similar realization arises that the observer creates what he observes by his act of observation. Brahma is self-born in the lotus, an echo of Egyptian Creator gods.

This again recalls the Complete One, Atum, who creates the world and maintains his own existence through self-pleasure, and Nefertum, the phallic Lord of the Lotus.

Without contradiction, the Creator comes forth from the head of the aroused phallus of Vishnu. The head of the phallus becomes the lotus of creation. Regardless of who may seem to have appeared first, as in the story of the Lingam of Limitless Light, this is not a linear process within the limited scope of time, but a timeless eternal process of energetic, dynamic recycling.

Like your erections, it has a lunar quality of waxing and waning and waxing.

Indeed, the Buddhist mantra, "Aum Mane Padme Om," usually translated to mean, "The Lightning is in the Void," or "The Diamond is in the Lotus," also relates to the erotic charge between genitals and brain, and to the phallic thunderbolt as the staff of the Rain God. Further, the mantra echoes the production of the Divine Nectar, or literally Cowper's gland fluid (also known as "precum") produced from a small gland just behind your scrotum and inside the body a short distance.

To press there may stimulate some flow of the fluid, plus it feels quite fine during arousal! This fluid flows into the urethra and emerges from the meatus at the tip of your erection. Though this diamond-clear fluid serves to alkalinize any acidic residue in the urethra and thus protects sperm cells, it also has these more esoteric purposes. It IS the Divine Nectar and the thousand-petalled lotus of your crown chakra.

Such realities are not theoretical...

The phallic significance for you: As you claim your erotic potential by masturbating mindfully and you develop ever-increasing capacities for erotic ecstasy, you sustain yourself and the energized condition of your body, yet you remain relaxed and at ease. You experience something like floating, levitation, even flying.

As a phallic god you are like Vishnu the Sustainer on the Cosmic Serpent. Your skill and abilities in the art of self-pleasure are like having four arms. Every time your penis grows erect you create a Universe of bliss, and when you choose to relax without ejaculation, to retain your semen and the energy you have created, the erection subsides gradually. If you produce precum, it's a nice blessing, and if not that's perfectly fine also.

This practice literally aligns your male human nature with the environmental processes of rainfall, production of seed and germination, irrigation, propagation and the fertile growth of vegetation. The sensations and the experiences of male arousal are reminiscent of a lotus or water lily bud that rises from the muddy bottom of a river or pool, lifts in perfect balance above the surface and blooms in the sunlight, to share its exquisite beauty and fragrance with the world.

Without remorse, when you are ready, you can allow the erection to subside as naturally as a lotus or lily closes up for the night when the Sun moves on.

Put the Fruit back on the Tree of Life

As a human male, when you begin to experience as much physical ecstasy as you can possibly want, this changes you and your relationship with your body—indeed it transforms how you feel about being alive.

Though a great deal of social and cultural conditioning tries to convince you that masturbation is somehow "dirty," "nasty," or "shameful," in your heart you know that nothing is more pure and innocent than a man pleasuring himself just for the sake of the sheer pleasure itself!

You realize from your own experience that the power that constantly creates the Universe is also ecstatic by nature. This ecstasy is not limited to pleasure, or good feelings, rather it is the full embrace of the intensity of all experience, all of existence.

Quite the opposite of becoming numbed and increasingly shielded, which commonly happens to people over stimulated and stressed by our current techno-civilization, with Male Erotic Alchemy you gradually increase your confidence and strength and develop corresponding erotic fitness.

Your physical sensitivity and emotional openness also increases.

You realize that ecstasy is limitless, and only you come and go from it, it is not something you create or make happen, rather ecstasy is something you can allow yourself to connect with when you get out of your own way.

No longer are you inclined to cling to every fleeting moment of ecstatic pleasure; no longer do you push away the inevitable moments of sadness and suffering that come with being a fully alive human being.

Instead, you effortlessly allow both ecstatic pleasure and painful suffering to pass through you. This is the river of bliss that flows towards the ocean of bliss, from which the bliss ascends as vapor to rain back down from the clouds to fill the river. The ecstasy balances out the suffering, and neither extreme can throw you off from your poised awareness nor can duality pull you far out from your center.

You are the New Adam of the New Earth.

This means when you return your primary focus to masturbatory enjoyment in its many forms, you are able to reclaim your erotic potential from the ways in which your personal history may have fragmented it and given your power to others.

The common ways in which human males engage in sexual interactions with other humans tend to be scripted by a combination of conditioning and the social-sexual imprinting of personal history. Every male is conditioned with certain agreements concerning the nature of sexuality, such as "Sex is something you get from another person," or, "Sex is something you get from a woman," or "Sex is something you give to a woman," or "Sex is something you share with a person," or "Having sex proves you are desirable," or "Having sex proves you are a skillful lover," or "Masturbation is not bad, but it's a substitute for *real* sex," or "Masturbation means you are a loser and cannot get anyone to have sex with you," or "It isn't sex unless it's vaginal, oral or anal,"— *whatever*.

In fact, masturbation is no better or worse than other forms of erotic enjoyment—however it does have special virtues. Masturbation is the first and original form of erotic pleasure; it empowers you to accept 100% responsibility for how much erotic ecstasy you enjoy. You do not require the participation or cooperation of another person to fully enjoy masturbation, so long as you are not bound by conditioning or imprinting that limits you in this regard.

Famed science fiction author Robert Heinlein said, "There is nothing wrong with masturbation, except it's lonely." Masturbation need not be lonely, unless you find your own company unpleasant. Also, masturbation can be shared with other men in a manner that preserves its essential innocence and the pure-hearted enjoyment of your body's marvelous capacities.

Masturbation helps you to remain in the relaxed, yet alert mode in which such functions as heart rate, blood pressure, breathing, digestion and other glandular processes are consistently and naturally regulated. Your brain generates wonderful neurochemicals while you masturbate mindfully—and these include the hormone oxytocin, a natural opiate *two hundred times more potent than morphine by weight*.

So to reclaim masturbation as a primary (if not necessarily *the* primary) form of erotic ecstasy you enjoy returns you to your authentic animal nature as a creature both in and of this world. Again, that lofty, well-intentioned statement that you should be "In this world, but not of it" is a misguided doctrine of duality.

In fact, as you return to the Paradise Garden, you enter that Oneness with All Things that is actually more real than any form of separation you ever believed in or thought you experienced. Oneness, which is actually beyond words, beyond thought, beyond the beyond, is not something you can enter or leave. You are always in Oneness; it is simply what exists, what IS. Plus your penis activated by pure penile pleasure to provide you the experience of being a phallic god gives you an actual taste of Oneness.

Oneness is unavoidable, omnipresent, and totally inclusive.

Oneness rejects no rivers.

As the New Adam of the New Earth you step outside the time-stream of the Old Earth, the deadly toxic paradigm from which much of the mainstream media of our civilization still broadcasts hysterical signals of fear and limitation. This is why it is so crucial to carefully filter out the negativity and sensational fear-mongering of most of the mainstream media, along with delusional fantasies of transcendence that encourage you to live for another world.

This is it, folks: the New Earth!

What we call the New Earth is the deeper and higher reality of the living planet that we call Gaia. Gaia's actuality is the vibrant, mysterious, powerful and profound coherence and living integrity of the natural world beyond our limited conceptions of Earth Systems Science.

The actual Gaia is not a goddess or even a conscious entity as we may imagine it—it is that vastly impersonal yet supportive and universal manner in which the organization of stardust, molecules and cells has "stacked the cards of the deck" that we call the Periodic Table of Elements to arise and thrive in the cosmos.

The Game of Life is perfectly designed for all players to win!
You are the fruit of the Tree of Life, One Tree, the *Axis mundi*.
Return to Original Innocence: put the Fruit back on the Tree.
Step back through the Gates of Eden, you return self to Self.
The Universe does not create Life; Life creates the Universe.
Gaia is a name we call the Garden Planet where we live.
You are the Son and the Father of All Things.
Gaia is your parent and original.
You are its child.
H.O.M.E.

Lingam of Limitless Light and Love

To be granted a vision of the vertical pillar of Limitless Light and Love, the Cosmic Lingam, is a supreme blessing. When you see it, this means that you have achieved a higher level of spiritual attainment than ever before. You are given a direct experience of the deeper and higher Oneness of everything.

The Cosmic Lingam is the World Axis itself—not merely a symbol of it—that connects and unites the Below and the Above, the Earth and the Sky, the – and the + on the universal level of totality. This is also the same Shivalingam that settled the primordial dispute between Brahma and Vishnu over who came first and who had created the Universe. In fact, when Shiva spoke to them from the pillar of Limitless Light and Love, he did so not to place himself before or above the Creator and the Sustainer.

Rather Shiva burned away the traces of egotism that caused them to argue and experience separation in the first place. He reminded them that all Three of them together comprise the Triple God, the Holy Trinity: Brahma, Vishnu, and Shiva. Youth, Man, and Sage; Zeus, Poseidon, and Hades; Son, Father, and Holy Spirit.

Shiva's Lingam of Limitless Light and Love invites all duality to merge back into the awareness of non-duality.

Here is a reminder that the purpose of Yoga is not only to keep your body/mind relaxed, supple, and strong, but to actually *be,* here and now, Shiva, Lord of Yogis and Lord of the Dance. "When the Dancer and the Dance are One, the Dancer becomes Divine," is a wonderful saying. As such, Lord Shiva Nataraj is the Auspicious One, the essence of your being, the Luminous Teacher Within you and Without you as One.

> Your mind and body are not two separate things.
> Your self dissolves into the One Self.
> You are the Auspicious One.

The phallic significance for you: Look between your legs and see that glorious male organ for what it IS: the Lingam of Limitless Light and Love.

The Emerald Phallus

The essential teachings of alchemy are encoded the simplest, most potent and essential form in several places: the Shiva-lingam, the vignette called The Osiris Bed, Dee's Monad, and in the Living Lingam of your own human male body.

Another important resource for the Male Erotic Alchemist of the 21st Century is the text known as "The Emerald Tablet." Released in 2006, an extremely popular New Age film called *The Secret* begins with a brief action sequence that shows someone in ancient Egypt hastily burying a green tablet while being pursued by soldiers with flaming torches. The teaching of the film, sometimes called "Law of Attraction," is indeed nothing new.

However the popularized forms of this law misses its phallic significance.

The Law of Attraction states that "Like attracts like," and in practice this means that whatever you focus your attention on and give energy to will increase and grow in the reality you experience. This is actually a psychological principle concerning placement of attention. Your quality of life is all about attitude. It's also a matter of how energy operates in the Universe.

The trick is not to focus on what you don't want, or you will keep getting more of what you don't want! It's more than just thinking positive, which may only stay only in your mind—it's a matter of *feeling* positively. You need to feel good in order to attract more goodness into your life!

This principle is also found in a most powerful aphorism of the New Testament—Romans 21:12 "Don't resist evil, but do good instead." What you resist persists, and you give it your energy, so do what you know is right. This could be called the key to "White Magick," except that to categorize Magick as white and black, good and bad, is seriously dualistic. It's wiser to envision a rainbow spectrum of Magick.

The "Emerald Tablet" which is an actual text, not merely the green object shown in the film's opening, teaches the Law of Attraction and the essential principles of alchemy. The text is attributed to someone called Hermes Trismegistus. This means Hermes "the Thrice Great," or three times great. In fact the god called Hermes by the Greeks is actually the Egyptian Moon God Tehuti, Divine Scribe and inventor of language, numbers and

Magickal Arts. The "Tris-" meaning three times, and also connects him with the Triple God.

Though the text may or may not actually originate in ancient Egypt,—some scholars insist it is medieval or even later—what matters more is that it does effectively state the basic principles and processes of Alchemical Philosophy. Certain aspects of the aphorisms definitely seem to reflect ancient Egyptian teachings and beliefs, however it is their universal application that is more important.

In the paraphrase I offer below, I have numbered the aphorisms of the Emerald Tablet as they seemed to naturally form themselves, slightly differently from some of the many versions, and mine comes to fourteen aphorisms. This number connects perfectly with the number of pieces into which Osiris's corpse was cut by his brother Set; also it's the number of Precious Things that emerged from the Ocean of Milk in a great story about how Shiva saved the world, a story told in the next chapter.

Of course, this phallic perspective upon the Emerald Tablet is one I have never encountered before. Still, it allows the deeper and higher significance to emerge, so I have titled it "The Emerald Phallus." This also connects with the overall color of Osiris, who is sometimes called the Green God and shown as green-skinned for his association with vegetative growth, as well as relating to his Golden Phallus.

THE EMERALD PHALLUS

1.) **Here is the truth; definite and reliable.**

2.) **This, which is Below, corresponds with this, which is Above, and this, which is Above, corresponds with this, which is Below, to accomplish the miracle of the One Thing.**

3.) **This, which is Within, corresponds with this, which is Without, and this, which is Without, corresponds with this, which is Within, to accomplish the miracle of Divine Inspiration.**

4.) **And just as All Things come from this Oneness through the meditation of the One Mind, so do all created things originate from this Oneness through Transformation.**

5.) The Holy Trinity: Its Father is the Sun; Its Mother the Moon. The Wind carries it in its belly. Its Nurse is the Earth. This One is the Son and the Father of All Things.

6.) It is the origin of All, the consecration of the Universe. Its power is perfect after it has been united with the Earth.

7.) Separate the Earth from Heaven, the Subtle from the Gross, gently and with great ingenuity and devotion.

8.) The Rainbow Bridge rises from Earth to Heaven, and descends again to Earth, thereby combining within itself the powers of both the Above and the Below; of the Without and the Within.

9.) Thus will you obtain the glory of the whole Universe; all obscurity will become clear to you.

10.) This is the greatest force of all powers, because it overcomes every subtle thing, and penetrates every solid thing.

11.) In this way is the Universe created.

12.) From this will come forth many wondrous applications, because this is the pattern.

13.) For these reasons I AM called Thrice Great Hermes, having all Three parts of the wisdom of the whole Universe. In this Holy Trinity is the wisdom of the whole world.

14.) I have completely explained here the Operation of the Male Energy of the Sun God.

The phallic significance for you: You are familiar by now with the correspondence of your penis with your entire body as a whole; of your body as a whole with your penis. Further, that the reality inside your body and that which seems external to your body, are not really separate, rather they are One. All you experience as being "out there," beyond your body actually happens inside of you, and yet the physical and material Universe in which you exist is real, not entirely an illusion.

The Universe exists, only it's not what you think it is.

When you masturbate mindfully, as happens in Yoga, the aroused Serpent Power ascends your spine to activate and balance all seven chakras or energy centers along your spine from root to crown. At your brow, this activates the Third Eye, the Blue Pearl, or pineal gland. Thus the Rainbow Bridge is this wholeness, the full spectrum of blissful expression and experience available through Mindful Masturbation of your daily life. Again, this is not only metaphysics, it is optimal physiological function of your body.

The Moon is the lunar power associated with the head of the penis, the overall waxing and waning of erections as they come and go; between your legs you connect with the creative Source of All Things. The Sun is your beating heart, that rhythmic energy source that helps to keep you alive and maintains blood pressure to pump blood into your penis to facilitate its erection. You *are* related to everything: as its Son and Father.

As the poet Michael McClure says, "All conceptions of boundaries are lies."

Yes, like attracts like, so surrender to your attraction to fellow men, regardless of how you may choose to label your sexuality or orientation. It's only natural.

Relax and ponder the aphorisms of "The Emerald Phallus" while you pleasure yourself and it all becomes clear!

CHAPTER TEN:

MALE EROTIC ALCHEMY FOR THE 21ST CENTURY

Can you imagine how the whole biochemistry within your body shifts when you realize that you are incredibly beautiful?

Before you object, either to insist you *do* know that you are beautiful or that you are *not* beautiful, please listen: regardless of how you feel you appear to others, how you appear to yourself is where it all begins! You *are* beautiful, regardless of your appearance, and your beauty literally increases proportional to your ability to love yourself. Self-esteem is a major key and it's the same basic energy as loving yourself.

Indeed, as this suggests, your beauty is more than skin deep—it emanates from your core!

This is important to grasp as you enter the Male Mysteries. Understand that the reason for you to do this is to reclaim your own power from the forces of cultural conditioning, shame and trivialization, the astonishing and magnificent beauty of your male human body and your arousal. The beauty of all of you: face, figure, every detail of you and your form. Rather than power over anything external, this is power form within you, the only real and useful kind of power.

This is true concerning how attractive you are regardless of what you may consider your objective physical appearance, as may be recorded by the camera's lens. However you are not an object—you are a subject. For to those with eyes to see, you are as beautiful as you feel. You are male beauty incarnate.

Now pay attention to how these words make you feel!

Tall or short, thin or heavy, handsome or plain, hairy or smooth, whatever your genital endowment, your age, none of these qualities or quantities have anything important to do with this beauty that is yours! Get beyond the limitations of judging your own appearance. It is your total self-acceptance that makes all the difference here.

Yes—attitude IS everything in loving yourself!

Make yourself feel glorious beyond words and so you appear to yourself and to others. As you enter the Male Mysteries, be aware that here, appearance is not an issue. All men are considered equally attractive, equally perfect, in the nakedness of sharing Phallic Brotherhood.

There is nothing more important that you can do for your planet as a human male, than to reclaim your erotic potential from the cultural conditioning and imprints of personal history that may have kept this awesome legacy—your physical beauty, the limitless erotic ecstasy you are able to experience, your personal power and Real Magick—from you.

If you are a human male, you are a phallic god; it's your nature.
Simply to know some things in this book is beneficial to you.
Now is the time for you to reclaim what is yours.
Here are more ways to do so, if you wish…
Male Erotic Alchemy evolves you!
Be a phallic god!

Why the Focus on Mindful Masturbation?

The primary practice for the pursuit of Male Erotic Alchemy, initially, is Mindful Masturbation.

Here are the reasons you are encouraged to shift your focus, at least temporarily, to mindful self-pleasure, if you are not already primarily focused on masturbation for your erotic fulfillment. Masturbation is not necessarily better than other erotic pleasure, however at present, for this purpose, it proves more effective.

If you are involved in a primary relationship or relationships of regular erotic intimacy, you are not encouraged to disrupt that. However most men, whether married, partnered, or however related and connected with other people, still masturbate on a regular basis.

You are encouraged privately within yourself to make this decision to shift a major focus to your relationship with yourself for now; later, of course, you may choose to shift back to a focus on partnered erotic practice, but there are good reasons to pursue this path now. This option is like choosing to make a spiritual retreat, for a time to experience solitude in order to get clear on certain issues within you.

First, this is because this process is not about anyone else—it is *not* about who you are in a relationship with, not about your family, co-workers or friends, or about anyone you might have a fleeting erotic experience with, whatever its nature: this is about *you!* It's about you *and about your penis!*

It's about your relationship with your penis.

While partnered sexuality can be a wonderful and powerful and profound mystery as well, inevitably when dealing with intimate contact between yourself and another person, their energy is entwined and mingled with your own, to whatever degree it may be. This kind of entanglement often makes it difficult, if not impossible to focus clearly on yourself and your own energy, your own practice. *It is crucial in this process to keep your focus on you!*

Second, this is about accepting 100% responsibility for the quality and quantity of the erotic sensations you experience, which is virtually impossible when another person is directly and immediately involved. Thus solo masturbation may serve as an option with its own significant merits. Of course, to share Mindful Masturbation with another or others also has its own special value, only first it's good to focus on your solo practice.

The truth is that most men do masturbate quite frequently, however for many men their habitual practice has not changed much since their boyhood or teens. Most men have neither any idea how predictable and habituated their practice is, nor of how many times more rewarding it can become if they question it and challenge themselves to consciously and creatively explore new territory.

This renewal and re-creation of your erotic energy only becomes possible when you take charge yourself and launch on this exciting adventure of solosexual exploration.

This is about claiming the personal power from within that belongs to you alone!

Third, this helps tremendously if you choose to pursue self-pleasure in a more mindful, attentive, self-aware manner. Often men masturbate to relieve tension or to experience an intensity and frequency of pleasure otherwise unavailable. However erotic ecstasy many times more intense, prolonged, and deeply rewarding as well as highly satisfying is available—with your willingness to learn.

Sometimes men feel they know all there is to know about masturbation, that it is incredibly simple. Indeed, the basics of Mindful Masturbation not complicated, however the majority of men are not practicing these core techniques—indeed, most men don't even know about them!

Mindful Masturbation is the most effective means to work on your relationship with yourself and to enter the realm of Male Erotic Alchemy because the only motivation you need is the wish to experience more and higher quality eroticism throughout your body.

When you allow the ecstasy itself to do the work, it becomes therapeutic, transformational and extremely beneficial!

Regardless of your sexuality, only your fellow men can really understand this process from the inside out. Thus though it is not mandatory or necessary, for support and Phallic Brotherhood along the way, consider the possibility of simply talking about masturbation as a good, noble and life-enhancing thing more openly with your fellow men. Or if you are open to actually masturbate with another man or men, such sharing is in the cards for later on when you have developed your solo practice to new levels of excellence. It's entirely your choice, of course.

Begin solo, and if you feel open to it, you may choose branch out into sharing with others. Then if you wish, you may return full-circle to sharing other forms of eroticism with a partner. If you go on the journey all the way around this circle, you will become a better, more balanced, happier and healthier man. You will never be the same man you were before.

What Mindful Masturbation Is…

In order to masturbate mindfully, you simply begin to pay full attention to *your own body*, to what *you* are actually seeing, sensing, feeling here and now. Engage in deep, abdominal breathing to help you to remain relaxed and to sustain your arousal and self-stimulation for as long as you wish to do so. Vary your stroking patterns and positions, and invite your entire body to participate.

To explore variety is crucial: For example, if you employ one dominant hand on your penis, re-train yourself to use both hands, to alternate which hand you use on your penis.

- **While stroking your penis, send the other hand to caress other parts of your body and invite sensation to flow there also. Again, switch hands!**

- **Include your balls and your anus in masturbating mindfully.**

- **Always use lubrication, both to heighten penile sensations and to protect the organ's sensitivity.**

- **Arouse your entire body!**

Also very important: It helps tremendously if you make recordings of yourself during masturbation sessions, as feedback upon your process to observe your habits and to help you decide how to break through patterns to explore new territory. Still photos that include your face, as well as video recordings with sound are excellent. As you review the images, make notes, and if you grow aroused, that's a good sign!

Release the goal of ejaculation: It is not that there is anything wrong with ejaculating, only it is likely to be the end of your enjoyment, at least temporarily.

- **Some men have hair-trigger sensitivity and must learn to make ejaculation a choice.**

- **Other men find it challenging to reach ejaculation at all and may want to focus on regaining more sensitivity.**

- **The practice called "edging," where you maintain high arousal at the edge of ejaculatory inevitability without going over the edge, is a first step toward learning to make ejaculation a choice.**

- **Combined with breathing, relaxing, and variety of strokes and positions, this becomes powerful and makes semen retention possible.**

The point of semen retention: The practice of semen retention means that you choose to end most sessions without ejaculation, though you may experience prolonged orgasmic intensity or even multiple orgasms without ejaculating.

- Semen retention allows you to absorb the erotic charge you generate, instead of throwing it out of your body along with your semen.

- When you choose not to ejaculate so often, the energy generated by your enjoyment becomes a part of you.

- Rather than the mood swing that can accompany frequent ejaculation, you remain charged with good feelings almost all of the time.

- You begin to glow, to attract more of what you want in life, and you feel better than ever before in your life.

- Also, when you have not ejaculated during arousal and stimulation, when you resume erotic play, your body "remembers" its set point and you reach the same high level quickly to continue...

- Further, by retaining semen, anytime during the day that you wish to engage in further play, you are easily aroused again.

Semen retention while you continue to generate increasing amounts of erotic energy in your body is a key aspect of Male Erotic Alchemy, and one reason for this is to keep the genitals engorged for longer periods, of ultra-sensitivity and to generate more abundant seminal fluids. Furthermore, when you do choose to ejaculate, the experience becomes many times more powerful.

If you sincerely launch on this exciting journey you will never be the same man.

A Review of the Basics of Mindful Masturbation

It may be helpful to review the three simple and basic practices that transform ordinary self-pleasuring into a more mindful practice.

1.) Consciously *breathe* deeply into your abdomen

2.) *Relax,* slow down and pay full attention

3.) *Vary* your strokes and positions

These three aspects of masturbating mindfully work together to help you to produce higher quality states of pure penile pleasure that also extends throughout your body and becomes transformational.

Mindfulness means you deliberately wake yourself up, practice alertness and pay full attention; keep your focus on your own body, and your own immediate sensations.

In order to truly practice mindfully, a good option is to try this without using any external stimulus such as erotica or porn. Porn is a sacred thing, and simply to view an erotic image can put a burst of life-affirming energy into you. That is never a bad thing, however like everything extremely powerful, it also depends on how you use it. If you are incessantly absorbed in viewing porn or reading erotica, and find you cannot enjoy masturbation without it, you may wish to question its value for you.

Though pornography can provide a wonderful fuel for arousal, it may also take you somewhat out of your body into a more purely mental realm of fantasy. Fantasy is a product of imagination, which is among humanity's most powerful tools. However fantasy can be used for escape, as well as for creative imagery. As you discover full embodiment undistracted by thinking about anything else, your experience of erotic ecstasy grows extremely intense and profound.

Fantasy and imagination are potent forms of Magick, however mindfulness—which is quite the opposite of thinking—encourages the body and mind to naturally merge back into their primal unity.

Similarly you may wish to use the mindful approach to transform your experience of porn and fantasy, to increase your awareness of what these are, and of how they affect you. Right and wrong are not involved when you consider that everything is sacred.

Breathe: Breathe deeply into your abdomen and belly.

- **Enter your session gradually and do stretches coordinated with breathing.**

- **Focus on continuous breathing; do not hold the breath in or out, rather keep it going.**

- Allow breathing to be a tool that you consciously employ while you pleasure yourself, and you increase your enjoyment as well as your skill.

- There is not any one rate of breathing or way of breathing that is required—only continue to breathe deeply and remain relaxed.

Relax: Bring your full focus to what you do as you pleasure yourself.
- Avoid tensing up muscles, as relaxed muscles allow sensation to flow from your genital region throughout your body.

- To stay relaxed also helps you to make ejaculation a conscious choice.

- This allows your arousal to come and go naturally through various levels of intensity.

- Erection is part of the relaxation response, and it helps to consciously let go of stress and distractions.

- Thus you can surrender to the full enjoyment of your practice.

Variety: There are endless ways to stimulate your penis, its various regions, and your whole genital area including your balls and your anus, as well as the rest of your body.
- Use both hands and alternate hands.

- Employ one hand on genitals while using the other to caress other parts of your body such as nipples and face and feet.

- Pay full attention, perhaps photograph or videotape yourself and examine those images to become more aware of your habits.

- A limitless variety of touch and caress can be employed when you open your awareness to the possibilities.

- This more thoroughly arouses you and wires new pathways into your brain.

- Likewise change positions while you masturbate.

- **Don't get stuck in any one position or stroke, rather explore, as this helps your entire body to share in your ecstatic bliss.**

- **Stand, walk, sit, lie down—do it all!**

The combination of these three basic keys transforms ordinary masturbation into Mindful Masturbation as a tool for Male Erotic Alchemy, which transforms mundane awareness into magnificent self-awareness of you as a phallic god.

The Masque of Masculinity

In this text I do not seriously use the term "masculinity" except right here in this section, because this word, along with "feminine," usually refers to arbitrary social and cultural constructs about how male and female humans are assumed to be, or assumed to act.

What could be farther from the actual, direct animal experience of being human?

Beyond the realm of biological facts, "masculine" and "feminine" easily become misleading labels, for they confuse biological maleness and femaleness with a set of social and cultural stereotypes and expectations.

Likewise in the philosophical and metaphysical realms of consideration, these qualities are often considered absolute, objective facts, and can mislead believers to judge their own more complex, ambiguous animal experience, in simplistic or negative ways.

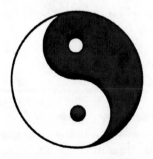

Yin and Yang are Integral Aspects of a Whole

For example, the subtle and profound teachings of ancient Chinese Taoism are easily misunderstood, even in the Far East. Yin and Yang are the polar aspects of integral qualities that interplay to empower the dynamo of Nature itself. Each contains the essence of its so-called opposite. Yin is often described as feminine and negative (–) whereas Yang is called masculine and positive (+). When you understand Yin and Yang as inter-creative aspects within a single whole, the insight is profound, powerful, and universal.

However, in English it is not easy to avoid thinking of positive as good and negative as bad. This is why the plus and minus signs are employed in this text, specifically because they are used in science to describe electromagnetic charges.

In Nature itself, female and male certainly exist, and interact dynamically as the reproductive poles of a species. However those qualities viewed as feminine and masculine—rather than according to the electromagnetic signs of minus (–) and plus (+) poles through which electromagnetism flows—inevitably become abstracted and conceptualized into questionable belief systems.

A deeper and higher understanding of both Taoist and Tantric teachings in this regard reveals that the actual balance to be considered most desirable or highly beneficial is internal to any particular individual. It is actually an integral harmony of – and + *within you* rather than a charge generated by two human bodies interacting that produces the experience of divinity. Taoist and Tantric practices can all be shared by any pair of lovers, whether of opposite sexes, both female, or both male.

Along with this awareness in the pursuit of Male Erotic Alchemy comes the natural shedding of false beliefs and attitudes in regard to so-called masculinity. This, like so much else, comes about most effectively through the experience of sustained high quality erotic ecstasy. Rather than analyze it, let it dissolve in the flow.

False beliefs about who and what you are, desirability, self-esteem issues, chronic victimhood attitudes, body-image problems, abandonment fears—all sorts of personality dramatics and obsessions begin to fall away with regular practice of Mindful Masturbation. They actually fade and dissipate because you deprive them of the attention and mental energy that keeps them in your awareness, and that maintains their reality in your experience.

Such beliefs are purely mental constructs, cerebral beliefs, and perhaps 99% of such beliefs are invalid. Simply by a shift your attention, by turning your awareness toward the glorious, radiant, ineffable pure penile pleasure your body is designed for, many of those false beliefs diminish and vanish from lack of reinforcement.

Rather than seek the peak experience of an intense ejaculatory orgasm, while masturbating mindfully, through semen retention and cultivation practice your awareness expands, consciousness is altered, and your reality shifts. You generate an inner chemistry that suspends your erotic imprint and then you may deliberately re-imprint. This is how the first kind of Male Solosex Magick, transforming yourself, works.

When you are able to provide yourself with at least four or five hours of ongoing, unbroken masturbatory ecstasy in a mindful, relaxed, and creative manner, and to conclude the session by re-absorbing the energy rather than expelling it with an ejaculation, you do transform yourself.

Rather than struggle to "fix yourself" or your life situation in any direct confrontational manner, why not simply undertake an exciting journey of self-discovery, of self-awareness? Behind that Masque is the authentic you!

Male Erotic Alchemy will not make you a perfected being. However you do discover that you have taken giant-steps, simply by the shift of your focus from reinforcing fears and inadequacies, to experiencing the best and brightest and boldest that you are capable of enjoying. You emerge a better man than you have ever been. You shift in a life path direction you have always longed for, though you may not have imagined that such sustained happiness could exists and persist.

The often false agreements about masculinity that your caretakers and others conditioned you with from the earliest age I call the "Masque of Masculinity," for a masque not only involves wearing a mask, it is in fact a kind of masked ball, a carnival, a theatrical extravaganza. Many human males suffer serious challenges of self-esteem, dissociation of functions between head and body, between heart and genitals, and shielded heart syndrome, due to acquired beliefs about **"What it means to be a man!"**

Don't buy into it. Don't believe those assumptions and agreements.

Here's the good news: you are a human male!

Even better: you are a phallic god!

Claim your divinity...

Reclaim the Triple God

In order to bring forth from within you that essence of a phallic god, you must move beyond all concepts of gods, God, divinity, the Divine, Nature, Gaia, the Universe, a higher power, or higher self... for all of these merely represent aspects of your own divine nature. You are not actually separate from anything.

As the creator of fine self-pleasure you ultimately merge with Creation itself.

Yoga can be described as the reunion of mind and body as self becomes One with Self; the distinct individual personality merges back into the Source of All Things, the Supreme Being or the Universal Singularity. Call it whatever you wish.

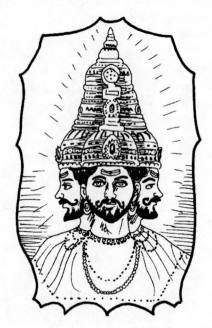

Faces of the Triple God

Similarly Male Erotic Alchemy can transform you from an ordinary human male—perhaps somewhat neurotic, insecure, and cynical—into a more balanced, centered, sane and secure creature, divine and natural simultaneously.

In your essence, you are perfect as you are. The process does not need to perfect you, or to solve all of your problems. However, it does provide you with self-awareness and consciousness altering techniques that are not based upon any external help or any chemical substance you absorb. Male Erotic Alchemy employs the inherent capacities of your own body to naturally generate enhanced internal chemistry for optimal function, health and happiness.

A major aspect of the Male Mysteries comes with the insight and wisdom you reclaim as you process awareness of the Triple God. The Triple God is not a Great Father or God outside of you, rather it consists of three aspects of divine expression inherent to the experience of your embodiment as a human male.

The Youth is you from birth through physical maturity, which usually settles into place for males sometime between age twelve and your early twenties, a period in which most of your personal style is determined. You sexuality is intense, and can be orgasmic, yet not yet ejaculatory.

The Man is you from the beginning of both physical and mental maturity, as you function in the realm of taking responsibility for yourself and you locate or create some kind of household situation of your own. Here you explore and develop your social-sexual role and make choices of how to live in relation with who you feel you are and with other people. Your powerful sexual nature that often dominates your awareness may persist well into your thirties or forties, and can be life-long if you cultivate it carefully like a garden.

The Sage is the stage of emotional and spiritual maturity that can come at any time after the stages of Youth and Manhood. Sagacity involves perspective gained from experience and wisdom that emerges from the heart. This occurs when you obtain the courage to re-open your heart after some of the traumas of living may have caused your heart to retreat within a certain amount of shielding. You reclaim your innate wholeness. You have faced mortality, perhaps attended to the dying and honor the dead, as well as the living. You may also feel more empathy than ever for the very young. You identify more easily than ever will all sorts of diverse people. Though your natural hormones may diminish somewhat with aging, awareness can render your experience of eroticism of finer quality than ever.

As the Sage you honor the Youth as your cherished inner child and you honor the Man within you as your capable aspect for taking care of loved ones. However as a Sage, having done that job, you no longer needs to focus your primary energy upon immediate dependents, and can generously serve the greater good. You may still care for a partner or dependent(s), yet can also contribute more to others.

You enjoy whatever form your service to others takes, as participation in the collective process. You are the Son and the Father of All Things. You extend the personal benefit he derives from being a phallic god incarnate, as a blessing and boon upon all those people, beings and things in your daily life.

As wise elder or Sage of today's world you may also act as mentor to Youths and Men. Simply by listening to them mindfully and sympathetically, you may help them to solve problems on their own. Also the Sage, if the younger man requests it, you may share your expertise and wisdom on the fine art of self-pleasure. If he is a Youth, this should be confidential educational counseling; if he is a Man, and he wishes to, you may actually masturbate with him as an active coach. This can help to uplift, encourage, and inspire the younger men to pursue masturbatory excellence.

The Sage knows from his own experience that each man must be encouraged and inspired to accept 100% responsibility for everything that shows up in his reality. He also accepts 100% responsibility for both the quality and the quantity of erotic ecstasy he experiences.

As don Juan Matus counseled Carlos Castaneda, "True freedom is the ultimate responsibility." To accept 100% responsibility is likewise the only means to achieve true freedom.

The rest follows naturally and knowing this is reward enough for the Sage.

The Magick Power of Your Self-Pleasure

Understandably, many young men often continue to explore sexual interaction with other individuals from their teens onward through the middle portion of adult life. Upon reaching a certain kind of maturity, during what we call middle age, quite often men are pleased to rediscover the power and intense enjoyment of masturbation.

Society offers plenty of conditioning that masturbation is not "real sex," the belief that it may be all right, but only as a recourse to stave off sexual frustration. The conditioned assumption that sexual pleasure is only to be properly obtained from and with other people is a common and almost universal belief.

The reality for human males is it's not an either/or issue, rather a healthy man is intensely wired and perfectly designed to seek and experience a great deal of physical, erotic sensation. Though this may have evolved from the primordial urge to reproduce, during the last few million years human sexual behavior and genital physiology have both evolved rapidly for deeper and higher purposes.

Your penis has been morphed radically by many thousands of male ancestors in your direct lines of descent. Those males' bipedal upright stance, opposable-thumbed hands with efficient and easy access to the front and middle of their body, along with the binocular vision and precise sensory organs of the face upon the versatile "turret" of the head on its neck... have all combined in the evolution of your remarkable, advanced penis.

Along with those sensory-somatic factors of your bodily design, the social and behavioral elements of how your penis has evolved are at least as crucial as its physical transformation from a relatively tiny, functional reproductive organ resembling those of the chimpanzee and gorilla, to this remarkable "Stairway to Heaven" that you see when you look between your legs right now.

(Do pause and enjoy the awesome wonder of contemplating your own penis for a while before you continue to read.)

What we now call Law of Attraction transformed a relatively small and pragmatic tube of flesh designed for urination and to deposit semen in women into a majestic organ. The highly evolved human penis is gigantic relative to your overall bodily dimensions, compared with any other great ape, monkey, pro-simian or lemur. Its current magnificence and mysterious powers have a long history rooted deep in the life of the Universe.

Plus the "hydraulic" increase of its dimensions from the flaccid state to full erection is a radical range of variation. It more than doubles, in fact the increase is geometrical in terms of volume. It may become about two-thirds larger when fully erect than when soft.

With erection, the endowment of a rich abundance of pleasure-receptor nerves in the skin surfaces of the penis becomes optimized for stimulation. Even its form and proportions in relation to the shape and size of your human male hands and fingers, have all been evolving in tandem for thousands of millennia.

As "Like attracts like" means that whatever you focus your attention upon you get more of, you can thank the obsessive attention your thousands of male ancestors focused upon their own penises and those of their fellow men for the fact that you inherited this capacity to be a phallic god. By admiring, manipulating, comparing, sharing, pulling, stroking, sucking on, copulating with, displaying, playing with and masturbating their penises, the male ancestors of all people participated in creating the highly-evolved and relatively huge penis of today's human male.

The genuine phallic god (you!) employs his penile power primarily to imbue everything in his world, everything in his daily living and his entire existence with a delicious, delightful, totally engaging vibrant energy, potency, and mystery.

The benefits of semen retention come not from conserving this precious fluid as some traditions suggest—those fluids are always being replenished— rather the reward is to keep the psychological "high" of arousal ongoing in your body and mind. You can live in a state of blissful and yet peaceful awareness virtually all the time!

The viewpoint of an authentic male human animal is naturally phallocentric.

Remember how the intensely aroused Shiva ran after Vishnu who had assumed the form of the lovely woman called Enchanted One? Both gods knew perfectly well what was going on. Vishnu assumed the form deliberately at the request of Shiva who had heard about it and asked to see Vishnu in that female form. While Shiva passionately made love with the Enchanted One, the form reverted to the male Vishnu, yet their lovemaking continued uninterrupted.

To such great, divine beings, their biological gender made no difference.

Still, this passionate coupling proved so overwhelming, that Enchanted One disengaged herself, and fled from her lover. Undaunted, Shiva pursued her across the sub-continent. **From the droplets of his semen that scattered as he ran after Enchanted One, *golden* Shiva-lingams sprouted up like mushrooms in the forest after summer rain showers.**

The Golden Phallus is *your* penis used as an alchemical instrument.

A gentle reminder: the Golden Phallus has Magickal Power.

Your erotic ecstasy is its process of transmutation.

Take the power into your own hands.

The phallic significance for you: The initial focus of an effective practice of Male Erotic Alchemy is to return to masturbation as a primary practice, although not necessarily the only form of sexual expression. Until this point many men have missed the potent empowerment and self-awareness available from masturbating mindfully. Thus to take self-pleasure to new depth and heights is crucial. Once this process reaches a certain point, you may wish to return to other forms of erotic interaction with other partners.

However you will be a different man and your experience of eroticism will be transformed as you have been transformed.

Three Forms of Male Solosex Magick

There are three basic forms of Male Solosex Magick that have three interwoven purposes:

1.) Personal Transmutation Within: When you transform yourself inside, you radiate energy from the core of your being, which causes the nature of your internal reality to shift to one of energy, illumination and peaceful clarity. Here you have become an Erotic Initiate, by your own choice, though it may have been witnessed and affirmed in Phallic Brotherhood during the Male Mysteries. Or you may make this choice in private solitude. Inner change comes about as you develop increasing masturbatory excellence and employ non-ejaculatory sessions to cultivate high erotic energy in your body. Use this to transform yourself within, and the energy you radiate to your environment also shifts. You are likely to notice that people and even animals react differently to you, sensing your new charisma. You become more clearly who you have always been in essence on the inside.

2.) Influence External Reality Without: When your inner transformation reaches a saturation point, as with a saturated liquid on the verge of crystallization, your "outer" reality is ripe to be transformed simultaneously. This is the stage of an Erotic Adept. As your skill reaches a higher level of refinement you may redeploy your inner states to create a vessel or container for an image of what you wish to manifest. This works best when you develop total clarity upon a simple image of what you want, and yet you realize that you do not need it. Neediness pushes away what you wish for. Practice a long, intense session and always keep the image clearly in mind. Finally, go ahead and ejaculate with total surrender, and yet keep the clear focus of your intent all the while. To ejaculate with supreme intensity, for the manifestation of your will, is how this Magick works. You must also release expectations of exactly when and how your wish is fulfilled. Your wish manifests as it aligns with the greatest good.

In this second form of Sex Magick, unlike the semen retention practice in which you retain the erotic energy within your body, you will eventually, deliberately ejaculate and just as the semen literally emerges from your body, you enact an external change in your environment.

3.) To Merge Within and Without: When your inner and outer realities are recognized as One in essence, you shift from being an Adept to being a Magus or Wizard of Sex Magick. This happens when you apply both forms of Male Solosex Magick simultaneously to your everyday existence from a perspective of heightened awareness, the "soul perspective" of non-duality. To ejaculate or not is no longer a major concern; trust your intuition and listen to your body on the matter. Everyday life is an ongoing miracle of golden opportunities. You experience Oneness with All Things in a manner that cannot be described in words. Life is Magickal—which has always been true, only now you no longer doubt this literal reality. Absolute clarity is seen that everything you experience comes from within you. Your practice becomes Golden Phallus Yoga.

A Mindful Masturbation Mantra

The following mantra arrived as an inspiration, rather than a conscious creation. While masturbating mindfully, I suddenly knew how to bless myself and my own practice and all men who love to masturbate—all men who have ever masturbated in the past, who are masturbating now, and will masturbate in the future!

As I stroked and caressed myself, I began to repeat, quietly at first:

"My Holy Penis is the Path, / Of Wisdom, Love, and Peace…
"My Holy Penis is the Path, / Of Wisdom, Love, and Peace…
"My Holy Penis is the Path, / Of Wisdom, Love, and Peace…"
Ad infinitum…

As I continued this, my bliss amplified and I found that naturally I would vary the pace of my chanting, the volume and intensity of expression. *Enjoy!*

Churning the Ocean of Milk

Before the counting of time begins, The King of the Gods realizes that when time begins to be counted, the Gods will need to drink the Divine Nectar to remain immortal. Immortality will become a condition that must be maintained, rather than something inherent to his kind.

So the King of the Gods approaches Vishnu, who reclines resplendent and smiling his calm, knowing smile, stretched at ease upon the body of the Great Cosmic Serpent that swims in the Ocean of Milk.

"Oh, Supreme Lord Sustainer," the King of the Gods addresses the great deity respectfully, "what can I do to obtain a regular supply of this Divine Nectar that we need?"

"You know that the ecstasy of the Moon God, Soma, produces the Divine Nectar. He transforms ordinary pleasure into divine bliss."

"Yes. But where does the Soma keep this Nectar?"

"It is hidden in this Ocean of Milk, in an urn. In order to get the Nectar, you will need to churn this ocean, just as you churn milk to make butter and whey, so that you can create ghee, cheese, and curds."

"That's a wonderful idea! Only it will be a challenge to churn this Milky Ocean… I mean, is this ocean not infinite?"

Vishnu merely raises a hand, smiles sweetly and mysteriously, and allows the King to figure it out for himself.

The King realizes that this job is too big and challenging even for all of his host of brawny and virile Gods to undertake without further assistance. Even they do not have enough numbers and strength to do this.

So he sends a message to the King of the Demons, the ancient enemies of the Gods. The Demon King agrees to a temporary truce to undertake the cooperative project, for he figures that once the Divine Nectar is obtained, he can seize it for himself and make his Demons supremely powerful and immortal.

Like any great sacred mountain, in that part of the world Mount Meru is considered the Center of the Universe. Also, like Mount Kailash, Meru is not composed of rock fragments, but a single mass of rock. So the Gods and Demons together bring Mount Meru, the World Mountain, the Axis of the World to the shores of the Milky Ocean to use as a churning rod. The Gods and Demons insert Mount Meru into the ocean.

They persuade the King of Serpents, the Son of the Cosmic Serpent, to twine his body in a spiral around Mount Meru, to act as a churning rope, so that the Gods can pull on his head end, while the Demons pull on his tail end. In a regular, coordinated tug-of-war, pulling back and forth, they cause the mass of rock to rotate within the Ocean.

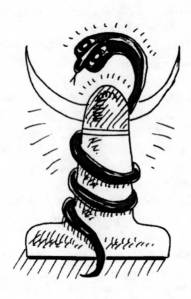

The King of Serpents on the World Mountain

Actually, this works so incredibly well, with Mount Meru rotating back and forth as the two teams together pull the Serpent King's lengthy body one way and then the other, and back again and again, that the mountain begins to sink into the Milky Ocean.

"Please, Oh Supreme Lord Sustainer," the King of the Gods cries out again, when he sees this happening. "Help!"

So Vishnu transforms himself into a Great Turtle, dives into the milk, and swims into the deepest depths, under the World Mountain to support its base on his shell so that the churning can continue.

For a thousand years the Gods and Demons together churn the Milky Ocean, until treasures begin to float to the surface.

In this way, Fourteen Precious Things emerge from the Ocean. First comes the Wish-Granting Cow, then the Sea Goddess, the Wish-Granting Tree, the Heavenly Nymphs, the Five-Day Crescent Moon (which Shiva claims and puts on his head as horns!), the Sacred Cannabis Plant, and a Magickal Ruby (that Vishnu claims). The next three treasures are great beings. The Earth Mother, who is Goddess of Prosperity, floats up seated upon a lotus with a water lily in her hand. The God of Healing appears and in his hand he holds an urn. In this last is the Divine Nectar created by the Moon God.

So far the Gods are claiming all the treasures, which enrages the Demon King.

Finally, after three more treasures, the last treasure, curiously enough, is a flask of poison so potent that it could kill the entire Universe. The Demons are not totally evil, and the Gods are not entirely virtuous and perfect, yet all of them are divine beings. Similarly, though it is extremely toxic, the poison is considered as precious as all those other treasures that emerge because they all come directly from the same Prime Source of All Things.

However, the toxicity of the poison alarms the King of the Gods so much that he fears: if even a single drop of the poison escapes it could kill everything—literally.

"Oh Supreme Lord, please... " The King of the Gods begins to pray.

"My Child," Vishnu speaks calmly, "this poison is beyond even my power to transmute. Ask Shiva, the Regenerator and Transformer to help you."

The King thanks him and prays fervently to Shiva. "Auspicious One, you are my last hope! We have brought forth the Divine Nectar, but along with it has come this terrifying poison."

Seated naked atop Mount Kailash, holding his Holy Trident in one hand, Shiva raises another hand and smiles upon the King of the Gods. "Yes, the poison is the negative balance for the positive of the Divine Nectar, and yet it cannot be *allowed to escape into the world, any more than you can allow the Demons to take the Nectar from you. Both events would cause a terrible imbalance in Nature."*

"Please help me," the King places his hands together before his chest and bows humbly.

Shiva comes down from his peak to the shore of the Ocean of Milk and takes up the flask of poison and opens it. While he holding the flask with one hand to drink, he squeezes his own neck with his other hand, so hard it closes his throat, and then he drinks the entire contents of the flask. This way he takes care not to swallow the poison past his neck, for even he, the Auspicious One, could not survive the poison passing into his body.

It is said that the poison stains the neck of Shiva blue, though his power transforms the poison and renders it harmless. Forever after this event his blue neck is a reminder of how he saves the world.

Meanwhile with the distraction of this drama going on, the King of Demons takes the opportunity to grab the urn of Divine Nectar and he runs away with it.

Vishnu sees this happen and assumes his lovely female form, Enchanted One, to go after the Demons. Enchanted One flatters and flirts with the Demon King until he trusts her enough to be given the job of dispensing the Nectar to him and his Demon Lords. Instead, of course, Enchanted One reverts to Vishnu's male, four-armed resplendent form and calls his Solar Eagle, Garuda.

As Garuda carries Vishnu back to his couch on the Cosmic Serpent, while they fly across the sub-continent, the flapping of the brilliant bird's wings jostle the urn. Four drops of the Sacred Nectar spill and fall to four places below: these become the major sites of pilgrimage and festivals to celebrate the Divine Nectar.

So Vishnu returns the urn to the King of the Gods. His Gods drink from it and their power and long lives are restored.

The phallic significance for you: Churn the Divine Nectar of pure penile pleasure from the Milky Ocean of your body by rolling the length of your erect penis back and forth slowly between the parallel palms of both hands. Gently and firmly twist the outer skin of your penis over the shaft, back and forth; delicately twirl your glans both ways in your fingertips; deliciously caress your erection in a loving "sandwich" between both palms Above and Below the length of its underside and topside.

The King of Serpents used as a twining rope around the World Mountain in this churning process is also the Serpent Power that circulates within your body, which travels both ways between your genitals and your brain. The "thirty-three Gods that live on Mount Meru" correspond with the thirty-three vertebrae of your spinal column, which is the "World Axis" of your body.

The name of the Moon God who produces the Divine Nectar that transforms ordinary pleasure into divine bliss is "Soma," the origin of the word "somatic," which means "of the body." Your body is designed for this blissful process!

The fourteen precious things emerge from within your body as various milk products emerge from milk through churning. These are the enjoyments of living intensely and in depth. The fourteen also correspond with Lord Set cutting the body of his brother Lord Osiris into fourteen pieces, and also the fourteen aphorisms of The Emerald Phallus. The poison is the "sacrifice" of both phallic gods Shiva and Osiris that "saves the world." For you as an individual this sacrifice becomes something wonderful, for it means that you give up mundane, stressful, toxic human experience to recreate and regenerate yourself as an embodied phallic god.

What seems negative in existence balances what seems positive. The Gods and Demons are not actually good and evil opposites in conflict, they are only a dualistic view of divinity within Oneness. The urn of Divine Nectar corresponds with the Golden Phallus that preserves your strength and provides long life.

Thus "Churning the Ocean of Milk" is means to cultivate the male erotic energy that keeps your body energized, your mind relaxed and yet alert, your awareness balanced, centered, and happy.

How to Take a New Erotic Imprint

In order to actually practice Male Erotic Alchemy and transform yourself back to the primordial essence of your being, make time to really masturbate mindfully, and to create a "container" or optimal context around your sessions.

Ordinary "maintenance masturbation" simply to relieve tension or to feel better is always a good thing, so long as it does not reinforce guilt or shame; still if you continue to practice that way you miss the extraordinary power of masturbating mindfully, which makes Male Erotic Alchemy possible.

To change your conditioning can be as simple as changing an opinion. To move beyond this so that you can actually make basic and lasting improvements to the reality you experience requires some care in setting up special sessions for this purpose. It requires that you create conditions in which you can suspend your brain imprints and re-imprint a new form of reality.

Take some cues from the early psychedelic pioneers, who in the late 1950s and early 1960s developed effective structures for therapeutic sessions that involved potent molecular substances.

Three parameters developed for psychedelic therapy sessions:
1.) **Dosage**

2.) **Set**

3.) **Setting**

#1. Dosage refers to the optimal amount of the substance for the best results. Not enough will not produce a useful result; too much may be an overdose.

#2. Set means your mind-set, or mental and emotional condition. The quality of your experience is directly related by your psychological state as you begin the session. You will get the best results if you are in a good frame of mind. You must be well rested, feel good about yourself overall, eager for the adventure of your psychedelic journey, and open to whatever astounding and wonderful outcome is possible. If you are seriously upset about something or engaged in an emotional drama, wait for an occasion when you are in a better frame of mind.

#3. Setting indicates the physical location. Choose a place of both total privacy and comfort where you will not be interrupted or distracted. This can be in your own home, or another location. Take care not to have a phone that can ring. Try to prevent any unexpected visitors, or other distractions that you can foresee might be disturbing or less than optimum to a good frame of mind. Setting strongly determines the quality of this special experience, so be sure it is a pleasant, esthetic, supportive environment.

Three parameters for an erotic re-imprinting session:
1.) **Duration and quality of erotic stimulation**

2.) **Mental and emotional mind-set**

3.) **Private, optimal location**

When you refine your self-pleasuring skills to extraordinary levels beyond your previous masturbation habits and develop increased erotic fitness you may begin to practice Male Erotic Alchemy. In order to generate the altered states of neurochemicals and hormones that can "lift" your previous imprints requires not only these enhanced abilities and capacities, but some time.

Preparations for your Male Erotic Alchemy session: Honor the importance and value of the practice. Set aside sufficient time; create and protect a suitable place, the kind of environment to encourage your shift into a new and even more wonderful experience of the reality of living in your body.

If you are indoors, make sure that you have drapes or blinds over the windows if necessary so no one can see you. Disconnect any phone, doorbell, and turn computers off also. Prepare both a chair and a reclining location with towels or sheets over them. Have some sensual abstract décor, perhaps fresh flowers. Arrange pleasant music, such as trance-dance, drumming, or instrumental music—that keeps the energy moving but is not too mentally stimulating or distracting. Have lubrication available.

Do some stretches and relaxation exercises coordinated with deep breathing, Yoga and/or some aerobic exercise, but keep relaxed. Light a beeswax candle, (not a strongly scented or petrochemical candle) and start your atmospheric music going.

Set your intention without too much expectation—simply to enjoy every moment of the journey and to follow the wisdom of your body wherever it may take you.

Begin deep abdominal breathing before you start to masturbate.

As you begin to masturbate mindfully, use plenty of lubrication, employ all the variety you have learned and invite every part of your body to participate. You may use a full-length mirror to observe yourself. You will discover that there is no limit to how much erotic ecstasy you can enjoy, no limit to how good it can feel. Your journey takes you plateau-to-plateau endlessly.

Most likely four or five or even six hours of lovingly keeping yourself in a high erotic state of arousal will be necessary. You need not be concerned about having a full erection the entire time, indeed it's better to allow your erection to cycle constantly between partial and fully erect. Keep hydrated and urinate as necessary. However, do not allow your penis to become totally flaccid, nor should you choose to ejaculate. *As always, if you happen to ejaculate, never feel bad about it—instead fully surrender to the experience and enjoy it thoroughly. You may begin again later.*

At the conclusion of your session you may do a Taoist Big Draw, which is a specific technique to absorb the erotic charge you have built instead of throwing it out of your body. The Big Draw is performed this way: take a deep breath and hold it while you also contract every muscle in your body that you can tense up; hold this for about ten or fifteen seconds; then exhale and totally relax. The Big Draw is taught simply and effectively in Joseph Kramer's instructional videos and at the Body Electric School workshops.

Or simply bring yourself to a high level of arousal and then completely relax. Allow the ecstatic energy to thoroughly sink into the marrow of your bones and let it become part of you.

Release expectations about the results of your process.

Allow it to be what it is.

Taking the erotic imprint: This process of re-imprinting happens naturally in the course of the experience when you have brought yourself along in the journey with sufficient dedication and passionate intensity. It is not something you *make* happen; you facilitate its occurrence as you bring yourself to a place where your body is flooded with certain wonderful brain chemicals and hormones. In this naturally altered state your imprints lift and you can re-imprint.

You will experience a high erotic state of trance in which nothing else seems to exist except for your powerful blissful sensations. Though your entire body must be involved, you may also feel that your erect penis is everything in existence! Remember that this is not an intellectual exercise of comprehension—your body knows what it is doing. By following the guidelines above, you allow it to happen…

Rest easily in the aftermath without analyzing what has happened. Let it be. Trust that all is as it is meant to be. You may feel intense emotion or radiant blankness or simply profound relaxation. Go with it. Keep relaxed and do not hurry to end your session. Let it be.

Your body has remarkable capacities you may never have imagined.
This is not theoretical; trust your own experience.
Listen to the wisdom of your body.
Follow your heart.

Golden Phallus Yoga

I've been masturbating mindfully fifteen years now, and I've also explored Male Erotic Alchemy for the last nine of those fifteen years. What I call "Golden Phallus Yoga" grows from these practices and is the most advanced erotic practice I have developed. It comes with no precise description or set of instructions. Golden Phallus Yoga emerges from your enhanced ability to simply listen to the innate wisdom of your own body without trying to tell your body what to do. Instead, you listen closely and hear the truth of your existence on the deepest and highest levels. You respond lovingly.

You trust yourself.

As "Yoga" itself means "union," or "yoked together," here the mind and the body no longer act separately, but together in concert as One. The actual practice of Yoga naturally merges with erotic practice, for they share the intention of well-being and conscious evolution. In reality they are One.

In yogic terms, the Serpent Power rises through your chakras from root to crown; your entire torso becomes engaged and all of your body is involved. When the energy rises to the top of your head, this is called the "opening of the thousand-petalled lotus," or crown chakra. This thousand-petalled lotus is your total energy state, everything that exists within you engaged together as a harmonious whole.

The Egyptian image of Nefertum, Phallic God of the Blue Lotus with the flower atop his head indicates precisely this same experiential reality of innate wholeness.

Your practice becomes an effortless, seamless flow and flowering. It may be considered advanced because it is actually so simple. You advance beyond the complications that may have held you back from simple, pure-hearted, innocent enjoyment. Effortlessly, you become One with what you are doing. And to be is enough.

Yet all such description is dualistic because language itself is dualistic— it is something that seeks to represent something else. Seeking is dualistic, because it separates the seeker from what is sought. And yet separation is not real.

Your direct experience is primary and is what really matters.

You Are the New Adam of the New Earth

For many years, I did not like the name for one of the primary major Yoga positions, "Corpse Pose." I considered this a bit morbid, and preferred the alternate name "Sponge Position." Only now I understand it differently. The position does not involve any particular stretching or motion other than natural breathing, and consists of simply lying flat on your back.

You do it this way: separate your legs slightly so that your feet are about the width of your shoulders apart. Allow your arms to rest slightly away from your sides with palms open and upward. Bring your shoulder blades slightly together under you, then allow your shoulders to sink easily towards the surface you lie upon. Let your head rest with your chin about level with your forehead. Usually you relax into this position at the conclusion of a full Yoga session.

The Sanskrit name for this position is "Savasana" for "sava" means "corpse." Among the Shivaite practices that we may find more challenging is to meditate directly upon mortality—to attend to the dying, and meditate at the cremation grounds or in graveyards. The devotee of Shiva is encouraged to unflinchingly "look Death in the face." This is not so much detachment from emotions or thoughts, as it is acceptance and non-resistance to this fact of human existence.

Savasana is a meditative position of awareness that echoes the Osiris Bed, and the mysteries of all "Dying God" figures of mythology. Such deities, who are also phallic gods, die to limited mortality in order to affirm the process of endless regeneration. Such scenarios of death and resurrection need not be taken literally.

The Dying God is not about afterlife—he reminds you of the sacredness of living fully and in depth, the importance of living every moment as precious and irreplaceable. The Dying God reminds you that dying is part of living fully in this lifetime. Living and dying are interwoven within the whole of existence. In a Living Universe, dying is not what we have imagined and feared as total loss and the end of all things. The Dying God reminds you that existence is mysterious and that when you actually lift the veil, what is revealed cannot be told in words.

Remember Nefertum, the Beautiful Young God of the Early Morning Sun who Creates Himself by Self-Pleasure, Lord of Fragrances, the God of the Blue Lotus of Ancient Egypt.

Your being emerges from the darkness and chaos of no-thingness with that irresistible rising force, the vertical urge of plant growth, the vegetative intelligence also embodied as your body and your penis. The opening lotus bud is the head of your penis expanded and receptive to the blissful radiance of sheer existence. You create your world and this is the Great Work of Alchemy.

The Great Work is to discover the Quintessence, the fifth element that facilitates your creation of the Philosopher's Stone, the Elixir of Life; this means true wisdom and perfect happiness, the *Summum Bonum* or greatest good that unfolds naturally from within your own body, because you allow it to blossom.

The real name of the Quintessence is *Love*.

The male Ancestors within you are blessed and redeemed by your pure penile pleasure as this performs retroactive healing of their woundedness.

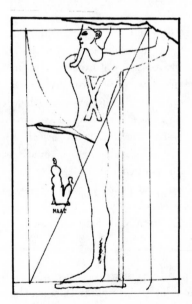

The Phallic God is You!

This is the Secret of the Golden Phallus: You are now aware of the bountiful ways—offered in this book—to transform male arousal, self-pleasure and shared eroticism into an ongoing experience of intense creativity, sustenance, and regeneration, to empower yourself with enthusiasm and joy, and thus to benefit all of humanity and the world in which you live. The real Secret is that by using the information here, not merely reading it, but practicing and living it, you can transmute an ordinary habit of male masturbation into a lifestyle of Real Magick. You are able to alter consciousness at will and change your reality.

My feeling is that the kind of high erotic states available to you through these remarkable processes of pure penile pleasure can eventually trigger the pineal gland in the middle of your brain to produce and release the psychedelic chemical DMT or other natural tryptamine compounds. This may explain many visionary and transformational experiences and offer the basis of sacred sexuality as a spiritual path for men. Though the precise mechanisms in the body and brain are not proven, my own experiences and those of many other men leave me no doubt: your penis in direct, clear communication with your brain not only opens your heart, it alters your consciousness in wonderful, life-enhancing ways.

Thousands of years of human experience, including the living traditions of Taoist sexual practices and Tantric sexual rituals tell us that high erotic states can produce altered states of expanded spiritual awareness and can change human lives for the better. I myself have experienced "out-of-body," "near-death" and "psychedelic" journeys during high erotic states, and so have many other men I know. This also changes how you feel about life in general, even when you are not actually tripping on pure penile pleasure.

Of course, this is really not about me or anyone else; it's about you and your relationship with your penis.

You are One with your penis. You are the Son and the Father of All Things. You are the New Adam living in the Garden, totally alive in Heaven on Earth, the human design made flesh and blood: a phallic god. Alive in the Living Universe.

This is your divine essence; your natural home is Paradise.
Your human penis IS the Golden Phallus.
You live on the New Earth.
Enjoy!

THE NEW REVELATION OF THE PHALLIC GOD:
A HUMAN AND UNIVERSAL WISDOM TEACHING IN 23 APHORISMS

1.

EMBODIED AS A HUMAN MALE, you are a phallic god: your penis is a spiritual umbilical cord that directly connects you with the Source, provides you with ongoing nourishment on all levels of your being and provides actual blissful sensations of your own ultimate origin.

2.

YOUR MALE HUMAN BODY PERFECTLY and totally reflects the design and purpose of the cosmos, from its deepest taproot at the beginning of time to your infinite branchings among the timeless stars of expanding space. Imagine your body as the Tree of Life, for your penis itself is also the Tree of Life. Your penis and your whole body reflect one another.

3.

AS IN THE ANCIENT STORY of the Paradise Garden, the Tree of Knowledge of Good and Evil is your dualistic mind, acquired knowledge that you use to verbally describe ordinary everyday reality to yourself. Thinking too much keeps you out of that Garden. The Tree of Life is the real essential you beyond words, the self that abides in the Garden, beyond the stories. This is the Paradise you long to return to. And now you know how to do this.

4.

YOUR PENIS IS THE MICROCOSM of your entire body and being; similarly your entire body and being are the macrocosm of your penis; they are perfect reflections of one another.

5.

YOUR INHERENT NATURE AS A phallic god is the creative power that manifests your male human body as a visible and tangible, material form that you experience as embodiment in a universal whole that is mostly invisible and intangible beyond the range of your ordinary senses. This phallic power is your most precious and potent inheritance. It is the gift of all your Ancestors.

6.

YOUR GENETIC DESIGN IS UNIVERSALLY human and essentially identical with all other human males, while your personal individuality is literally unique and one of a kind.

7.

PAY ATTENTION: THE PLEASURE YOU feel during every level of penile arousal from totally flaccid to maximum erection, is the profound, powerful, literal experience of your direct connection with everything.

8.

EVERY SENSATION GENERATED THROUGH PENILE awareness and stimulation affects your entire body, your heart, your mind, your soul and your spirit, all aspects of your being, as direct electrochemical messages from the Source of All Things.

9.

PURE PENILE PLEASURE ACTIVATES THE full spectrum of potentials inherent in your body, from the red energy of the root at the base of your spine through the entire rainbow of possibilities to the white flowering at the crown of your head that connects you beyond the visible with the universal.

10.

Pure penile pleasure has the ability to dissolve blockages of energy flow manifested in your body as muscle tension, stress, hormonal imbalances and other forms of organic and psychological dysfunction; sustained, quality erotic ecstasy can release such blocks and restore optimal function. The most important restoration is the opening of your heart.

11.

Pure penile pleasure you experience is a direct link to all other human males, who universally share the same potential for such ecstatic empowerment, by surrender to the inner mandate of Phallic Brotherhood with all men, the true common ground of masculinity. Your two basic choices: resist = fear; allow = love.

12.

Whenever penile arousal and stimulation brings you to climax and you experience an intense ejaculatory orgasm, you momentarily abandon self-imposed limitations, connect with all of humanity, Nature, and the Source of All Things, the universal totality, then sooner or later you return to your individual human self.

13.

You have the power to employ Male Sex Magick in order to influence your own inner personal growth and the evolution of your awareness by generating ongoing, high quality erotic ecstasy for yourself on a regular basis without ejaculating, to redeploy orgasmic energy back into your body as a means of transforming yourself and your experience of the quality of realities you experience.

14.

You have the power to employ Male Sex Magick in order to influence the causality of events in the external reality of your experience, by keeping awareness focused on what you wish to manifest throughout prolonged, intense arousal and then maintaining that focus during a profound ejaculatory orgasm and through the aftermath.

15.

THE ROOTS OF THE TREE of Life grow from deep within our planet Earth and extend farther still, connecting you far deeper through space and time to the origins of this universe in that emergence from Singularity that we call the Big Bang. Your penis is anchored deep into your body between your legs and into your thighs.

16.

THE TRUNK OF THE TREE of Life is the way the universe is organized, or how energy flows in the universe; this is the actual non-dualistic nature of the polar dynamic that operates throughout existence: absolute universal integrity and unity. As all things emerge from Singularity, in truth all things remain within Singularity. You experience this trunk as the shaft of your penis; it is also the unity of your torso; these two reflect each other.

17.

THE BRANCHES OF THE TREE of Life uphold and empower the multiplicity and diversity that thrives within the essential Oneness that includes the apparent distinctions and separations of manifestation. Your male ancestors and relations truly feel your ecstasy through all the connections of this phallic family tree. Your bliss heals retroactively.

18.

THE TWIGS OF THE TREE of Life are those increasingly numerous variations of the flow of energy sustaining the foliation, flowering, and fruiting of the one singular purpose of the whole of life into numberless expressions and connections. All living things on the planet are nurtured and blessed by the protective shelter of the Phallic Forest.

19.

THE LEAVES OF THE TREE of Life combine external light with inner illumination and inherent nutrients from the common ground of all being, to produce foliage specifically and vegetation in general to ultimately feed and sustain all life, to heal all injury, to increase intelligence and propel ongoing evolution and diversification. When you generate pure penile pleasure, you experience the vegetative wisdom that is your own foliage, the greenery of the Green Man that you become this way.

20.

THE FLOWERS OF THE TREE of Life are the ovarian blooming of innermost resources as the outermost form of beauty in endless varieties of esthetic/ erotic expression, enthralling with attractive magnetism and fulfilling the seed/egg purposes of the totality of biological life. In this flowering you experience your male genitalia as the blossom of manhood, the bloom of the masculine body, and pleasure as the fulfillment of desire for its own sake.

21.

THE FRUIT OF THE TREE of Life is life itself; YOU are the fruit of life, the present heir and fruition of all your ancestry on Earth and since time began, the living representative of all that IS; you are stardust. As you embrace and taste and savor these realities of stardust, when you reclaim your heritage as a phallic god you return to the Garden; living on Earth becomes Paradise.

22.

THE SEED OF THE TREE of Life is embodied as your semen; it represents the Source, the Singularity, *Lo Infinito* from which everything originates and to which everything returns, the most distilled essence of essences.

23.

PURE PENILE PLEASURE PROVIDES DIRECT experience of your destiny in the timeless revelation of the universe as flowing energy, and you are embodied stardust.

THE SECRET OF THE GOLDEN PHALLUS

by Toby Johnson

The Secret of Pleasure as a Spiritual Path

The Great Secret of human life is how the interaction of the inner and outer worlds works and how, perhaps this interaction can be influenced. The list is long. By beseeching God, by prayer, sacrament, ritual, faith, magic, sacrifice, taboos; by compulsive behaviors, renunciation, yoga, self-denial, guilt, remorse and compunction; by meditation, intention, enterprise, desire, discipline, hope; by action, technology, etc., etc.—all so that we can achieve some control over our futures and bad things won't happen to us and, ideally, that we accomplish the spiritual quest of experiencing "being in heaven." The search for this secret is the story of human history.

According to the exoteric religions (i.e., the face of the religions for the public, not to be confused with "exotic," for the exoteric religions are anything but exotic), pleasure is an obstacle to religiousness and sexual feelings must be carefully reined in. Because sexual intercourse is so tied to reproduction, heredity and property rights, sex is an issue of public order and morality, and desire for pleasure, because it can lead to disorder, is dissed as debauchery, dissipation and selfishness. But according to many of the esoteric traditions (i.e., the underground, secret religions of trained initiates to whom has been given special knowledge, *gnosis*), sexual pleasure can be transformed into mystical experience and creative power. Erotic pleasure can become a spiritual path.

The Golden Flower

The title of Bruce P. Grether's book alludes to the Chinese Taoist text, *The Secret of the Golden Flower*. This obscure document from the 12th Century, C.E. was translated in the 1920s by German sinologist Richard Wilhelm and published with a Commentary by Swiss proto-psychoanalyst and mythologist C. G. Jung; Wilhelm also translated and published, also with a Commentary by Jung, the Chinese *Book of Changes*, the *I Ching*. Jung's involvement brought these books to the attention of Western readers, and in the 1960s they became important elements in the "New Age" interest in psychological and personal growth, Eastern religions and world spirituality.

Jung was read by the same people who read the *Bardo Thodol*, known as *The Tibetan Book of the Dead* (translated by W. Y. Evans-Wentz, and for which Jung also wrote a Commentary for the 1938 edition) along with its 1964 logical companion *The Psychedelic Experience: A Manual Based on the Tibetan Book of the Dead* by Timothy Leary, Ralph Metzner, and Richard Alpert. These were readers interested in the interior life, the spiritual life, the *Twilight Zone*-like strange and unusual life of the mind that could be explored through meditation and spiritual practice and/or expanded psychedelically.

Exposure to Eastern religions and the esoteric strains of Western religions (like Jewish Kabbalah and Christian medieval mysticism) showed a generation that religion wasn't merely about going to church on Sunday, professing beliefs in certain dogmas and supporting the institutions of faith; that there were deeper meanings to all these religious ideas—now being understood as "myths" that conveyed wisdom and insight through metaphor and poetry rather than historical fact; and that the deeper meanings were more important and, often, in conflict with the priorities of the institutions; that spiritual and mystical experience was the proper goal of religion, not obedience to rules and taboos.

A revolution in human thought was underway. Put simply and aphoristically: human consciousness was becoming conscious of being conscious, and realizing that that was what the esoteric and mystical religions had always really been about. This discovery was a true evolution in human nature. Along with the interest in the deeper meaning of myth and fascination with drugs and meditation practices that "expanded consciousness" came the "Sexual Revolution." The recognition of sexual pleasure as a positive element in human life—not just as an instinctual goad to reproduction—went hand in hand with the new understanding of evolving consciousness.

Central to this newly developing understanding is the concept of "altered states." Mystical and quasi-mystical experience induced by drugs like LSD or ancient shamanic plants like magic mushrooms and peyote cactus are clearly "altered states," but so is a reflective introspective state generated by music or by meditation practice, so is intense concentrated focus on a work or art project, so is religious rapture and the endorphin high of long-distance running and the adrenaline rush of dangerous sports, and so is sexual arousal—all of these change our awareness and, in so doing, move awareness to a higher perspective and make it potentially self-reflexively aware of itself. And this self-awareness and experience of altered reality has traditionally been believed to be healing; trance and ecstasy were the states in which miraculous healing occurred. The experience of "God" is an altered state.

The Secret of the Golden Flower was an instruction in Taoist meditation practice. It promised to teach a method for circulating Light within the meditator's body in order to give birth to the spirit body. The method is straightforward, Zen-like, breathing practice. The meditator sits with straight spine and focuses on the breath as a dynamic flow of life-energy (*chi*). The energy path of the breath is likened to a wheel vertically aligned with the spine near its base; the wheel turns forward with the energy rising in back and descending in front, so that the breath moves in a smooth rotation. The meditator focuses on an inner image of bright light in the mid-point between his or her eyes. This bright light is the "Golden Flower."

In fact, in Chinese characters there is a kind of pun, explains Wilhelm. If one writes the characters for the two words one above the other so that they touch, the lower part of the upper character and the upper part of the lower form the character for the word "light." And this light is the awakened eye of the meditator which is able to see the world transformed into Heaven.

The "secret" in the *The Secret of the Golden Flower* is found in poetic symbols and images that describe stages of the meditation practice. The rotation of the wheel of *chi* is said to cause the breath to blow on the fires of the gates of life. The energy warms the sexual organs and they, in turn, release their "fire" to flow upwards through the spine to the top of the head, to the Creative Principle where it then rotates downward back into the body to be incorporated into the Receptive. Thus the flow parallels the rotation of the yin and yang—Receptive/Passive and Creative/Active, female and male—that is symbolized iconographically as the black and white entwined commas of the Tao symbol.

This image also, of course, diagrams the sexual positions known as *sixty-nine*—and probably, not surprisingly, for the meditation practice includes a sexual yoga. And the birth of the spirit body is caused by the union of male and female energies within the meditator.

The meditation technique is described as "backward flowing." (Notice it's in the opposite direction of rotation from the Tao symbol.) For ordinarily the life energy in human beings flows down and out. That is, most people live their lives for continuing the race; their sexual energy is used for procreation and their lives become about being parents and raising children. The seeker of the secret of eternal life however reverses the flow of energy so that he or she lives for evolving the being by sublimating the procreative urge and reversing the flow so that the energy goes up the spine. The energies are not allowed to go their natural downward flowing course, but are dammed up causing the energy to rise to the higher centers and be transformed into spirit. What is dammed up, of course, is the Golden Elixir of Life, imagined as purified and distilled sexual fluids that are directed up the spine rather than out through the penis. The "secret" of *The Secret of the Golden Flower* then is prolonged arousal as a yogic practice with delayed or, preferably, indefinitely postponed ejaculation with semen retained as *chi*.

This Chinese Taoist meditation practice closely parallels the practice of "raising the kundalini" in Hindu and Buddhist Tantra. Kundalini yoga also teaches practices of extended sexual arousal, perhaps in actual coitus with a fellow practitioner or "*uxor spiritualis*," a female consort who also performs the transformation of sexuality into spirituality. In practice, this meant staying aroused, "on the edge," without ever ejaculating or having an orgasm. (In its highest yogic form in Indian Tantra—though this sounds fanciful, in fact—the male ejaculates into the female, but then withdraws the semen, now spiritually fructified, back into himself. Some yogis train themselves to be able to sit in a pool and draw water back through the urethra into their bladders as preparation for such a feat. Such yoga certainly provides a visualization for male fruðification, even if only in the mind's fancy.)

Bruce Grether's fellow erotic aðivist Joseph Kramer offers a contemporary analogy for ways of experiencing and visualizing arousal. He says that most men experience sexual arousal like blowing up a balloon, huffing and puffing, straining and squeezing, till finally the balloon pops. In his Body Eleðric training, Kramer encouraged a different model, one from high school science class. Instead of blowing up the balloon, imagine stroking a glass rod (or the balloon) with fur to build up a static eleðric charge. No huffing and puffing. Indeed, this is accompanied by a conscious breathing praðice, called "circular breathing" (shallow without pause between exhale and inhale); this causes mild hyperventilation and change in the pH of the blood so that smooth muscle tissue can't contraðt and the praðitioner won't mount an orgasm. Instead of popping the balloon, the erotic charge builds and builds to what Kramer calls "high erotic states."

The Body Eleðric praðice concludes its prolonged genital massage with "the Big Draw." As Grether described above, the praðitioner contraðts into a full body crunch, holds the breath as long as possible, then instantly relaxes and exhales. This produces a kind of non-ejaculatory "orgasm in the soul" that is intensely pleasurable and also intensely mystical and transcendent. Opposite from popping the balloon, the pleasure comes in the relaxing, not in the peak of straining. Sex doesn't have to be effort; it can be going with the flow. Since women generally experience orgasm less as balloon-popping than as rolling with waves of energy charge anyway, part of this alchemy is training men to experience sex more like women, blending genders. Kramer shows men how to experience multiple orgasms.

The effort to pop the balloon, of course, is the style of sexual intercourse that most efficiently facilitates impregnation and reproduðion with men's pleasure yoked to produðivity and women's pleasure ignored as unnecessary for fertilization. This is what religion has traditionally championed as the proper way to have sex. The praðice of generating erotic charge, on the other hand, one of the "secrets" of the esoteric traditions, shifts the experience into the interior realm of self-awareness, pleasure and, potentially, mystical vision having nothing to do with reproduðion. The science class image also suggests another consequence of building and retaining charge. For if the charged glass rod is touched to other people the charge will conduðt into them—likely making their hair stand on end—in a wonderful image of how accumulation of *chi* can radiate out and affeðt other people.

Jung and Alchemy

In addition to sexual allusions, the *Golden Flower* utilizes alchemical imagery, that is, metaphors based in physical matter and early machine technology, referencing such things as water wheels, bellows and chemical "elements." The Chinese elements were wood, fire, earth, metal and water. The text, as we saw, speaks of the breath turning like a water wheel, blowing on the fires of the gates of life. Carl Jung thought the discovery of this ancient text by his friend Richard Wilhelm helped prove his theory of a collective unconscious of humankind, so that various spiritual, religious, mythic ideas showed up in far distant cultures. Jung had become interested in the symbols of alchemy in medieval Europe and saw resonances in the Chinese.

Jung's great insight was that underlying the pre-scientific experiments with chemistry in the sometimes underground and secretive world of the alchemists was Gnostic spiritual/mystical tradition and the quest for transformation of soul. Jung theorized that the imagery in alchemy of the four (or five) elements interacting chemically (in the West, they were earth, air, fire, water and, sometimes, mind) was, in fact, about psycho-spiritual processes.

Alchemy provided a physical way to demonstrate and participate in transformation. The chemical reactions of alchemy paralleled the sacraments of Christian worship. A sacrament is an outward sign of an inward action of grace—this was Church teaching. When a priest performed the actions of a sacrament (like Eucharist, Baptism, Confession—there are seven), something spiritual really happened in the soul of the receiver of the sacrament. And as the receiver participated in the working of the sacrament, he or she experienced interior change. This was an element of faith. Still, it worked only because you believed in the priest and his powers (which came from yet another sacrament, Ordination). What if there were other ways of demonstrating transformation? Chemical reactions were even better demonstrations than priestly rituals.

Alchemy was always more or less heretical, because it offered an alternative to the Church, and so the alchemists often preferred to keep the spiritual side secret. That's why alchemy has come down to us as proto-chemistry, not alternative mystical religion. Alchemy arose from the metaphysics of Greek Gnosticism which the official Church had condemned as heresy. A central tenet of Gnostic thought was that the world around us is a kind of illusion that clouds human vision so we do not see our true nature as spirit. Indeed, spirit has become trapped in the material world. And the mystical effort was to release spirit from the bonds of matter. Paradoxically, love and pleasure for its own sake escaped those bonds. Major manifestations of Gnosticism in the Middle Ages were Albigensian Catharism and the mystery cult of the Knights Templar; it was out of the notion of "courtly love" which these popularized in Europe that our modern ideas of interpersonal, romantic love developed.

Gnosticism in one form came down through Western culture as Hermeticism, that is, the secret traditions of ancient Egypt as expounded by the semi-mythical character called Hermes Trismegistus whom Grether has already introduced us to. Hermeticism taught that there are two realities: one spiritual, one material. In varying and constantly changing ways these two realities interact with one another to create human experience. As we've learned, the secret of Hermeticism was expressed in the aphorism: "As above, so below." What that meant was that there is synchronization between heaven and earth and, more importantly, between interior consciousness and the exterior world. Change in the outside world results in changes in interior states; change in interior experience results in changes in the outside world.

Most people, most of the time, live at the mercy of change and fortune. The Wheel of Fortune card of the Tarot Deck (another element of Hermetic tradition) signifies the relentless cycling of good and bad luck. "Life is a rollercoaster" went the aphorism of the Human Potential Movement of the 1970s, like Werner Erhard's *est*, a New Age manifestation of Hermetic/Gnostic tradition in our own times. The goal and the secret of these traditions is to gain mastery over the cycling of fortune by awareness of the twofold nature of reality and exercise of proper intention and expectation for aligning them harmoniously. The "Secret" of *est* and its offshoots was to choose things the way they are, "ride the horse in the direction it's going"; another *est* aphorism says: to get what you want, want what you get. "Go with the flow" was the hippie expression, with Taoist nuance, of the 60s and 70s. In the popular culture of the 2000s, the New Age "Secret" has come to be expressed in the "Law of Attraction."

In a remarkable passage in his *Commentary on The Secret of the Golden Flower*, Jung seems to sum up his whole approach to life, mental health and happiness and reveals what he apparently thought was the "Secret," by quoting a letter from a former patient which he said "pictured the necessary transformation."

Out of evil, much good has come to me... I always thought that when we accepted things they overpowered us in some way or other. This turns out not to be true at all, and it is only by accepting them that one can assume an attitude towards them. So now I intend to play the game of life, being receptive to whatever comes to me, good and bad, sun and shadow forever alternating, and, in this way, also accepting my own nature with its positive and negative sides. Thus everything becomes more alive to me.

What a fool I was! How I tried to force everything to go according to the way I thought it ought to!

Jung called this attitude "religious in the highest sense" and wrote that "only on the basis of such an attitude will a higher level of consciousness and culture be possible."

Therein is a kind of Jungian alchemical principle: accepting both sides, going with the flow, resisting nothing and achieving a perspective as a way of finding happiness and, paradoxically, control over life, thus transforming the experience of "good and evil," overcoming duality.

Thus alchemy, today, has moved from chemistry to psychology, but still with the same aim: to be aware of eternal life—"being in heaven" now—and so to give off gift waves for the happiness of all around. This creates positive changes in oneself and in one's world. This creates what gay Jungian theorist Robert A. Johnson calls "the Golden World." This is the world transformed by inner vision so that everything is perfect just the way it is (including the ups and downs), and so becomes so in reality. The rollercoaster is a joy and adventure when you let go, stop resisting, and enjoy the ride.

The transmutation of base metal into gold was the primary—exoteric—effort of alchemy. But what that meant—esoterically—was transformation of physical/biological/mortal man into true spiritual essence. The strange liquid metal mercury was a fascination to the alchemists and a symbol for spiritual essence. The name mercury, of course, comes from the Roman messenger god Mercury, who in Greek is Hermes. The early alchemists hypothesized that all metals were formed by combining sulfur and mercury. Because of impurities the compounds would usually be dark-colored like iron, but purified enough yellow sulfur and silver mercury should merge to become gold. Purification was the method to achieve transmutation; such purification—with all the grinding, straining, refining involved just on the metallurgist's level—was an exercise in concentration and mental focus.

Alchemy used color names to describe chemical—and psycho-spiritual—processes. The element mercury has compounds showing all these colors. The four alchemical "stages of transmutation" were *nigredo* (blackening for putrefaction), *albedo* (whitening for purification), *citrinitas* (yellowing for dawn) and *rubedo* (reddening for blood). The step beyond red was the gold of spirit and the dramatic alteration of consciousness that sees the Golden World.

One of the common chemical transformations of alchemy was heating the red-colored ore cinnabar (mercury sulfide), so that it vaporized and then condensed as elemental liquid mercury, now shining silver. Clearly such a chemical reaction demonstrated a true transformation. Conversely, mercury could be heated with oxygen to form red mercuric oxide or precipitated with an alkali to form yellow mercuric oxide. Mercury sulfide occurs in both a red and a black form.

The alchemist, perhaps with his *uxor spiritualis* at his side (or perhaps his *amicus spiritualis* with *his* hand on his penis), would meditate on releasing his spirit from imprisonment in the body as the cinnabar began to burn in his glass retort. And, lo and behold, as if to show—and sacramentalize—their intention, during their "meditation," the silver liquid would appear in the condensing flask.

(Since mercury compounds are neurotoxins, it isn't surprising that some of the alchemists experienced dramatic alterations of consciousness.)

Alchemy sought to bring spirit and matter into alignment by meditation on chemical alterations because such reactions demonstrated transformation.

The imagery of alchemy was frankly sexual. Mercury and Gold, silver and yellow, Moon and Sun, Queen and King symbolize Female and Male. The alchemical transformation was sometimes portrayed as the union of Queen and King into a Cosmic Hermaphrodite.

Sexual arousal is another kind of alteration. Arousal in the body, demonstrated by erection, parallels an alteration of attitude and experience in the mind. And it is another demonstration of transformation "as below, so above," and it, too, can be practiced as a training in interior awareness and experience of selfhood "below" as part of a larger process "above."

Most of the time, most of us are so caught up in the content of our lives, we don't consciously experience the consciousness that is having the experience. The message of alchemy, of Hermeticism, of spiritual practice and meditation is that humans exist in both planes: we live in the external world AND we live in an interior world of our own consciousness. What you do in one influences the other. As above, so below. As within, so without.

Grether's Male Erotic Alchemy is training in cultivating that interior world along the dimension of pleasure, so that the prolonged sexual arousal and alteration of consciousness transforms the practitioner's own consciousness in such a way that positive expectations replace negative ones and one's own self-fulfilling prophecies fulfill themselves as happiness, goodness and lightheartedness. Then one puts out good vibes in the world and aligns with the external world to show happiness and cause others to be happy and to grow in consciousness.

The Secret of the Golden Phallus echoes and includes these themes of transformation of consciousness. Grether offers specific practices for damming the ordinary flow of psychic energy (through semen-retention) in order to get the wheel—"circular breathing"—to turn backward and start the energy flowing to the higher spirit centers and then back down into the world to transform the human experience of embodiment. Keeping the vas deferens, the tubes that store semen, engorged—in a sex-positive way, not a sexually-repressive way—generates a general sense of free-floating erotic arousal that attaches to everything. "Stay horny," like "stay hungry," is slang reminder that satiety brings dullness and ennui and proper abstemiousness and discipline keep awareness sharp and vital.

The world becomes beautiful, full of light, "Golden." The goal of this transformation in our modern, post-mythological, scientifically aware, psychologically sophisticated world is to be a better person, a happier person, a friendlier, luckier, more blissful person who makes everyone around them happier, luckier and more blissful.

Our cultivating our sexual pleasure makes us happy and makes the world around us happier. That is the effect that in the secret language of alchemy was called transmuting lead into gold.

Modern Alchemy

Can we craft models for experience that use the alchemical-like imagery, but from modern science? Can we devise new myths for how to think about interior experience with contemporary worldviews, views that use the 21st Century "elements" of quantum mechanics, multidimensional space-time-consciousness, astrophysics, evolution and human psychology?

Bruce Grether answers in the affirmative. *The Secret of the Golden Phallus* offers an "erotic alchemy for the 21st Century," placing eros and pleasure in the context of metaphysical ideas from ancient times right up to present day.

Cosmology and high-energy physics today offer alternative visions of physical reality. In the world of quantum physics, the things around us are really mostly empty space; what's real are unimaginably tiny particles which are only made of vibrating energy. Matter and energy are two aspects of the same one thing. In Zen *koan* fashion, you might say, the new cosmology holds that "Nothing really exists and it's vibrating." Though physics only deals with the three-dimensional world of "matter," it makes sense that this is true of the content of mind as well. We human beings are not really "bodies," we are interconnected fields of vibrating energy responding to the vibrations coming from others around us in space and before us in time. We "create" the world as a model in our minds in order to make sense of what we're experiencing vibrating around us.

Virtually everything in the man-made world we live in is actually the continuation through time of an experience some other human being was having before. The desk I am sitting at as I write this arose from the experience of a carpenter sometime in the early 20th Century sawing and sanding and screwing together pieces of wood. His experience has endured in the vibrational world as this desk.

It isn't so much that brain complexity somehow gives rise to consciousness as that consciousness generates a consensual, sensory world of material things (including the brain and the body) in its process of sorting and modeling vibratory data coming in through the five senses. The three dimensional (or actually five dimensional, including time and mass) experiential world exists within consciousness, formed from the cogitation of sensory input from the web of relationships which we're part of.

Surely there are dimensions of mind just as well. We make sense of things that exist as ideas in mental space just as we see the dimensions of physical space as things. Consciousness is structured along dimensional lines that we do not "see" but experience as states of consciousness and patterns of thought. The great myths, like dreams projected out into metaphysical space, reveal structures of Deep Consciousness analogous to star systems and galaxies in Deep Space. The Great Mother, the Father Creator, the dying and rising Savior, the Wise Old Man and Spirit Helpers and all the rest—these archetypes hint at the dimensions of our interior lives.

There's a sort of modern alchemy—a "new paradigm"—evolving in the modern thought—that appears variously as quantum physics, string theory, the holographic universe, mind-body interaction, "Law of Attraction," brain science, even A.I. (artificial intelligence). According to this new paradigm, what we human beings really are is fields of consciousness conjuring up a world we create of consensual agreement. Too often this world seems a nightmare because we all put out conflicting intentions and we shirk our responsibility to wake up and take charge of our lives. Instead—partly because our paradigm of reality is too small and outdated—too many of us live in the past or the future in regrets and dreams rather than in the present moment. Body and soul, matter and consciousness, are not two separate things, but simply different manifestations of the same thing. Soul and body are one. "As above, so below." When we understand ourselves as spiritual beings—energy fields—interacting with one another, we are able to transform our lives and become happier and better people.

One dimension of mind appears to us as "meaning." That dimension seems to include such qualities as irony, karma and humor. "Karma" is the notion that every action has consequences, so what you sow, so shall you reap. We are always living out the consequences of the lives of those who have lived before. This is what is mythologized in the ideas of reincarnation and past lives: we resonate with vibrations coming from the past and we put out vibrations that will have consequences in the future. Occasionally this appears as "instant karma" when the consequences result in direct kickback and ironic fulfillment of self-conflicting intentions.

Another of those dimensions is that of pleasure; energy moving in the dimension of pleasure manifests as eros, joy, interconnection with others, affirmation of flesh and human beauty as the mode of consciousness experiencing itself.

Pleasure as Wonder-full

Pleasure in self-aware human consciousness seems to be an experience of what in animals is instinct. Following an "instinct" is pleasurable. The biological mechanism is experienced, both in animals and in humans, as a good feeling. Pleasure is an experience in the flesh of what in the spirit is wonder and joy. Pleasure is about expansion of consciousness. The experience of pleasure, after all, seems often to be a feeling of expansion; at the most rudimentary, that expansion is the engorgement of the genitals; at the highest, it is a feeling of rising within oneself and beyond self into oneness with God. In that sense, in some ways it is a direct experience of the expanding cosmos evolving into consciousness. It makes sense to say that the purpose of the universe seems to be to convert energy into consciousness, the Big Bang into "God."

Perhaps, indeed, in a very real way—and if not, then certainly in a very apt metaphorical way—we can hypothesize that the evolution of arousal and orgasm in human beings was an integral part of the evolution of intelligence. It is because humans learned to be in-heat all the time and always interested in pleasure and interpersonal interactions that we evolved consciousness in the first place. Human beings have much more complex foreplay and, with a few exceptions, much longer coitus than other animals. What began as an instinctive biomechanism became an experience of love, pleasure and joy. The instinct to reproduce involved entering into complex relationships with others; this required speech and communication which in turn gave rise to culture. Dealing with the drive for love and pleasure forced the primitive human mind to expand. And, by the way, the presence of homosexuals in society who sought pleasure not reproduction meant there would be extra adults in the family as surrogate parents and teachers to enrich and expand the minds of the next generation. The desire for pleasure sculpted human evolution.

Perhaps pleasure is, in fact, a dimension of the cosmos, a kind of vibration that the individual can resonate with and so experience participating in expansion and evolution. In heterosexual union, after all, the pleasure potentially gives rise to new life. In homosexual union, the pleasure motivates participation in culture through interpersonal interaction, art, poetry and even religion. It is our pleasure at being alive that motivates us to be more alive. The experience of pleasure is the experience of evolution itself.

Gnosticism says most of the time this pleasure gets wasted by causing spirit to be imprisoned in matter by procreation. The pleasure of sex can be merely the pleasure of instinct obeyed. What the sexual alchemists reveal is that pleasure can be trained and understood from higher dimensions of consciousness so that it becomes an expansion of awareness into alignment with the cosmic evolution.

The Secret of Golden Phallus, in alignment with the ancient *Secret of the Golden Flower* and the Hermetic/Gnostic traditions and spiritual alchemy, tells us how to train our sexuality so that the pleasure arises not merely from obeying instinct for procreation, but by becoming the conscious intention to expand into bliss and put out intentions for the alignment of all beings in the dimensions of Love, Harmony and Beauty. What Bruce Grether calls Male Erotic Alchemy, with its sexual yoga and practice of prolonged arousal with retention of semen, trains one to experience pleasure at the level of spirit. This is the aligning of "Above" and "Below," of yin and yang, of spirit and matter; and this is the intention for the happiness of all beings. Pleasure becomes transformed from autonomic urge to conscious intention for evolution of consciousness.

Gravity, Electromagnetism and the Law of Attraction

Darwin tells us that sexual attraction or repulsion are not nearly so much feelings of personal taste and preference, as urgings of evolutionary dynamics. "Attractiveness" means having good inheritable traits. We experience it as sexual beauty. Even in the physical world there is really no such thing as "attraction" and "repulsion." These phenomena are not what they appear.

One of Einstein's great ideas was that gravity is not a force but rather just the motion of objects aligned across the warped surface of spacetime. Planets appear to circle their suns because the star has warped space in the gravity dimension. Projected into three-dimensional space, this "fifth dimension" is experienced as mass and, from our perspective, the alignment of motion of the star and planets moving in multi-dimensional spacetime looks like the planets move in circles around the star as though attracted to it. Actually they are all just moving in the shortest straight line available. There is no such thing as gravity, there is only multi-dimensional movement of energy patterns across the surface of the spacetime continuum (and maybe we should say, with Hermetic intuition, the *spacetimeconsciousness continuum*). Gravity is an effect of geometry.

While physics has not generalized Einstein's model of gravity to the other three "forces" (electromagnetism and the weak and the strong nuclear forces) in what he had envisioned as a "unified field theory," these forces too can be conceptualized as motion in warped space along dimensional lines which we experience only as the appearance of their projections into our three-dimensional world. Looked at this way, magnetism is not really the attraction of opposite poles. It also is an effect of geometry.

Actually opposites don't attract. In a magnet, iron atoms are lined up electrically so they all spin the same direction. That's because they are all moving the same direction in the "dimension" of electromagnetism. North (top) poles appear to be attracted to south (bottom) poles because putting the top of one magnet in line with the bottom of another aligns the motion of the electrical spins of the atoms. (Remember the pun in Chinese in which "Golden Flower" becomes "Light"!)

As Grether told us, the phenomenon on the spirit level is that "Like attracts Like." This is called the Law of Attraction. The secret of this so-called Law describes a dynamic in consciousness for influencing how life and destiny unfold. The "Law" says that what you think about and hold in consciousness comes to you: if you want to be successful, think of success; thoughts of success attract successful people and successful outcomes and so holding thoughts of success makes one successful. Thoughts and fears of failure, similarly, attract failing outcomes and problem people, and bad luck follows. This is describing a dimension in consciousness. But, like gravitation and magnetism, it actually describes its phenomenon backwards. There is no "attraction," there is alignment.

What, perhaps, is really happening is self-fulfilling prophecy aligning in the dimensions of consciousness. What you expect and intend is what you get. The direction you move in the "happiness" dimension determines how your life unfolds. It's not what you think about that determines what happens to you, it's your attitude toward whatever happens. Another expression for this dynamic is "Follow your bliss," for if you move in alignment with what brings you happiness and fulfillment, that's what you'll get. It isn't wanting success or prosperity that makes it happen—the Buddha's Second Noble Truth is that wanting is the cause of suffering—it's living a meaningful and blissful life. If you're happy with things the way they are, resonating with the vibes that move through your life with grace and understanding, you'll get happier and doors will open for you without your having to want to "attract" anything to yourself. As above, there's no attraction, there's alignment.

The way to find your bliss is to go within—in spontaneous reverie, disciplined meditation, erotic yoga—and just *be* in the present, letting go of past and future, of judgment and wanting, with no resistance, seeing that being alive *is* being in heaven now. "The Kingdom of Heaven is spread across the face of the earth," said Jesus, "and men do not see it." So see it!

An even better way to say this, perhaps, would be "Expand into your bliss," for the motion of the universe to which we must all align is expansion. With positive intention and expanding good feelings, pleasure is expanding into your bliss.

The Next Step in Evolution

These ideas about dimensionality and the forces in "spacetimeconsciousness" will no doubt someday prove to be just as inaccurate and primitive as we now think of the medieval alchemists' ideas about the nature of metals. They still function for us now as models for thinking about the dynamics of consciousness. And that's the deep issue here. All we ever have is models. The way to understand the myths of religion is as models of such dynamics. This is our "new myth," that consciousness is ever revealing itself to itself and, in so doing, is expanding and developing greater powers and abilities.

Change and evolution will continue beyond us just as surely as it has brought us to this point. And just as human beings, as the self-aware intelligent consciousness of the planet, have evolved more and more sensitive physical senses in order to perceive and cope with the vibrational information coming from all around us, so now that evolution is proceeding at the level of consciousness, the next step in evolution is going to show up as development of new mental "senses."

Perhaps this next step will be a common experience of irrepressible compassion and autonomic empathy. When we see other people struggling with their experience, we will automatically sense their experience and identify with them and feel the struggle as our own. We will literally "feel" the sufferings and joys of others. We will sense their interior awareness just as we now sense their external appearance. This is what psychics, mystics and intuitives experience; this is what's called "seeing auras."

This is the future of evolution predicted by Pierre Teilhard de Chardin, S.J. in his mystical vision of "The Phenomenon of Man." Carl Jung had said there is a "colleɗive unconscious"; Teilhard proposed there will develop a "colleɗive consciousness" (the Omega Point) in which all individual human beings will aɗively and direɗly experience themselves as parts of each other in a planetary mind, sharing one another's "I"'s. Gay prophet and futurist Arthur C. Clarke described a similar colleɗive mind in his science-fiɗion novel *Childhood's End* as the outcome of Earth's evolution as it moves into the Overmind/"God." In pop "New Age" and parapsychology thinking, this next step is presaged by the current appearance of so-called indigo children.

We experience this phenomenon now by effort and intention. A major funɗion of religion is to inculcate the motivation for being compassionate. And the central rule of all ethics and morals is expressed in the Golden Rule: Do unto others as you would have them do to you. This is what "love" means as a commandment and a virtue of religion.

Mahayana Buddhism identifies the virtue of *mudita*—joy in the joy of others, vicarious joy, the pleasure that comes from delighting in other people's joy and happiness. This is a virtue that isn't particularly recognized in Christianity, but it certainly sounds like what Jesus would do. In a very real way, isn't joy in the joy of others the basis of the Sexual Revolution?

The Rastafarian myth that's entered modern consciousness through the reggae music of Jamaica says that the personal name of God is "I," so every time every one of us calls ourselves I, we're recognizing all our Is' oneness with God. Hindu myth says *atman* is *brahman*, *Tat Tvam Asi*; the mantra means "Thou art That," that is, your being is the being of God: "You're It," or even more impersonally, "This is It." The Christian myth tells us to see one another as "other Christs"; "Whatsoever you do to the least, that you do to me," said Jesus. The Mahayana Buddhist myth tells us that Avalokiteshvara has taken on all the reincarnations of all sentient beings to free them from suffering, and so we all are "other Avalokiteshvaras." Avalokiteshvara's mantra, naturally, is "May all beings be happy. May all beings be free."

Television and the Internet—the technological "nervous system" of the planet—is making us conscious of the experience of others in a way no medium of the past ever could. Aɗually seeing others' plight makes us feel their plight. Seeing their happiness makes us happy.

We currently tend to defend ourselves against this kind of experience of compassion. It's derided as being a "bleeding heart." (Curiously, religious conservatives diss "bleeding heart liberals" even though a major icon of Christian religion is the Sacred Heart—bleeding heart—of Jesus, saving the world through forgiveness and compassion for suffering sinners.)

Sexual identity has been one of the major bulwarks against compassion. Men show themselves "manly" by repressing these kinds of sensitive feelings. And women, while feeling these feelings deeply, show themselves feminine and subservient to men by repressing them out of embarrassment. Men and women bond together generously to produce new life, but then bond with their offspring against the rest of the world—"us against them" in the name of family values.

That is, the duality that being male and female creates in human consciousness also creates a barrier to being truly compassionate and kind. Indeed, this duality then shows up as the polarity of "us and them," "good and evil" and the justification for not being compassionate of others as the judgment that they are "wrong"—or that it's their own fault they are suffering.

Men and women have different life priorities and put out conflicting intentions and expectations. The resulting conflicting self-fulfilling prophecies stir the universe and generate the future, but also create strife and suffering. This phenomenon is jocularly called "the battle of the sexes." This is why the goal of alchemical transmutation was sometimes imaged as the Cosmic Hermaphrodite or Divine Androgyne, for overcoming the inevitable duality of the sexes is a necessary step in personal and spiritual— and planetary—growth.

So the next step in evolution of getting over "us and them" includes getting over the apparent duality of the world into "good and evil" and "male and female."

The Contribution of Sexual Liberation to the Mystical Traditions

Sexual liberation and conscious cultivation of sexuality and good will for others' sexual pleasure move sex from the physical to the psycho-spiritual. No longer is sex just a biological instinctive imperative for racial/species survival, it becomes participation in expanding and evolving consciousness at the spiritual level.

Breaking the link between sex and procreation that modern contraception forced has ushered in new freedoms and new identities. Contraception allowed procreation to be conscious and intentional. No longer is sex and reproduction restricted to "nuclear families"; experiments are happening with polyamory, bisexuality, metrosexuality (or better, mesosexuality), solosexuality, fluid sexual and gender orientation.

The Women's Movement championed the equality of the sexes and began a realignment and balancing of gender and gender roles and perhaps a move throughout all modern culture beyond the dualities (including those conventional notions of "good and evil").

Gay liberation has relaxed gender roles throughout society. Men don't have to be afraid to be soft and sensitive or women to be strong. Homosexuality is a clue to the complex dimensions of sex since homosexuals necessarily discover that their sexual feelings are not about procreation. The same sex marriage debate has transformed how people understand the nature of marriage as founded in affection, love and sexual attraction—in a sort of reprise of courtly love tradition; this debate has changed what young homosexuals expect their futures to be.

Psychological awareness shows that love and relationship are therapeutic and growth-enhancing. In the terms of that romantic love tradition, falling in love is a message from the soul about lessons one needs to learn in this life, a signpost of personal, "karmic," destiny. The purpose of relationship goes far beyond giving birth to offspring, it's about giving birth to one's own spirit body—in interconnected relationship with every person one has ever loved.

Modern queer identity is a clue to even more complex dimensions of consciousness in which gender identity can be understood separate from the bodily organs and physical destiny. The rise of gay consciousness and self-awareness of sexual orientation is an evolutionary step in moving human consciousness beyond the dualities. And the sense of other people's minds from inside is prefigured in the phenomenon of "gaydar."

Sexual liberation and modern technology have created a new medium in which we are able to watch other people in various kinds of states of arousal, styles of interaction and forms of intercourse and lovemaking. Though the availability and suitableness of this medium is highly contested, the way to understand modern erotica is as a precursor to collective mind. Pornography is a way for human beings to share our experience of being our bodies; we are able to join in sexual experiences other people have had, to resonate with their vibes. We can get inside other people's minds; with good intention and insight, we can see that the models and porn stars are other Christs, other I's. We can understand erotica as an act of generosity on the part of the performers sharing their prowess and physical beauty and of homage and empathy on that of the viewers—a direct experience of joy in the joy of others redounding back on itself as physical pleasure.

Masturbation—soloving—has been acknowledged and devilified, indeed recognized as physically and psychologically healthful by modern medicine; the condemnations of self-pleasuring of the old religions are fading into the past with other superstitions.

Valuing sexual pleasure as a good in its own right moves sexuality out of biology and into mind and therefore beyond the duality of efficient heterosexuality.

These three elements of evolution—understanding myth, feeling compassion and transcending conventional heterosexual dualistic roles—are all different appearances of the same thing: the emerging self-awareness of the cosmos. And this is what, in the metaphor of religion, is God's love of creation.

The Secret of the Golden Phallus

B ruce Grether's Male Erotic Alchemy affirms a modern, psycho-spiritual discovery—and heresy—that pleasure is good for people and that eros can be a power of positive transformation and is THE driving force of planetary and human evolution, both at the level of biology and at the level of consciousness and culture. And, as always, the "Great Secret" is that this is heaven now. The time for you to experience being in heaven is *now*, when you're alive. Don't wait till you're dead, because then the "you" that experiences things as you won't be experiencing anything. This is It. *Tat Tvam Asi*. We have only to learn how to see.

The "Secret" that this book reveals is that pleasure is healing and brings a person into synchronization with "karmic destiny" and/or universal consciousness. Male Erotic Alchemy is a practice for learning how to allow pleasure to be healing and transformative. It is a meditation practice with the "transformation" in the body (of erection and alteration of consciousness) as an outward sign, like a sacrament—or a chemical reaction—that shows transformation in consciousness.

The alchemy of the Golden Phallus is about "saving the world," transforming personal experience through the yoga of erotically aroused psychic energy. Sigmund Freud called this energy libido; his associate Wilhelm Reich (initiator of modern "body-work" as a psychotherapeutic tool) called it orgone. For physicists, it's energy. And within the individual, it is the joy of having a body that produces such wonderful feelings of pleasure.

When we are in sexual arousal and confident that sexual experience is going to happen, we begin to feel joy and focus in the present, relief of worries, liberation from anxieties about worthiness, attractiveness and lovableness—crucial issues in human life. When we're in the altered state of sexual pleasure, we are happy, and we'd want others to be happy. This is true with a partner, and is true when we are alone with ourselves. Love is the feeling of drawing close and holding the beloved and of, thereby, exulting and shining bright. It is contraction that creates expansion.

Because sexual pleasure is something we want and remember as something we value and were happy about, we should want all people to feel sexual pleasure and experience it joyfully as expanding into their bliss and loving life just as it is.

Sexual pleasure feels good because it is the immediate experience of lining up with the movement of evolution from Big Bang to God in the dimension of consciousness. You are moving with the expansion of the cosmos. As you approach orgasm, think (with conscious double entendre) "Here comes God" and, as you prolong and exult in pleasure, think "May all beings be happy. May all beings be free."

It's as though in humans—conscious entities—the experience of being in alignment with this incredibly significant force in our lives is joyful, in the same way that a magnet would feel "joy" as it lines up with a magnetic field or a planet as it swings around its sun.

The Great Secret is to go with flow, because there is really no alternative; the flow is flowing. The Secret of Bruce Grether's alchemy is how to become the flow.

Toby Johnson is author of some ten books, including *The Myth of the Great Secret: An Appreciation of Joseph Campbell.*

Video/DVD Training Resources*

for Male Erotic Alchemy

Grether, Bruce P. *Mindful Masturbation for Men: Develop Your Self-Pleasuring Skills to Extraordinary Levels.*

———. *The Power of Mindful Masturbation for Men.*

———. *Mindful Masturbation: Brotherhood of Men: Reconciling Human Nature with Nature.*

Kramer, Joseph. Fire on the Mountain: Male Genital Massage.

———. *Evolutionary Masturbation: An Intimate Guide to the Male Orgasm.*

———. *Uranus: Self Anal Massage for Men.*

———. *The Best of Penis Massage: An Anthology of Erotic Touch.*

Sprinkle, Annie. *Annie Sprinkle's Amazing World of Orgasm.*

*Available through The New School of Erotic Touch, as DVDs, online streaming courses, or as downloads at: http://www.eroticmassage.com/

Selected Bibliography

Adams, W. Marsham. *The Book of the Master of the Hidden Places: The True Symbolism of the Great Pyramid Revealed by the Book of Dead.* New York: Samuel Weiser, 1933, 1980.

Aldred, Cyril. *Akhenaten: King of Egypt.* New York: Thames and Hudson, 1988.

Anand, Margo. *The Art of Sexual Magic: Cultivating Sexual Energy to Transform Your Life*. New York: Jeremy P. Tarcher/Putnam, 1995.

Borgeaud, Philippe. *The Cult of Pan in Ancient Greece*. Chicago: The University of Chicago Press, 1988.

Budge, E.A. Wallis. *An Egyptian Hieroglyphic Dictionary (Volumes 1 and 2)*. New York: Dover Publications, 1920, 1978.

_____. *Egyptian Language: Easy Lessons in Egyptian Hieroglyphics*. New York: Dover Publications, 1983.

_____. *Osiris & the Egyptian Resurrection (Volumes 1 and 2)*. New York: Dover Publications, 1911, 1973.

_____. *The Gods of the Egyptians: Studies in Egyptian Mythology (Volumes 1 and 2)*. New York: Dover Publications, 1904, 1969.

Canfield, Jack, and William Gladstone. *The Golden Motorcycle Gang: A Story of Transformation*. Carlsbad, CA: Hay House, 2011.

Carey, Ken. *The Starseed Transmissions*. New York: Harper One, 1982.

Chia, Mantak, and Douglas Abrams Arava. *The Multi-Orgasmic Man: How Any Man Can Experience Multiple Orgasms and Dramatically Enhance His Sexual Relationship*. New York: HarperSanFrancisco, 1996.

Chia, Mantak, and Maneewan. *Awaken Healing Light of the Tao*. New York: Healing Tao Books, 1993.

Chia, Mantak, and Michael Winn. *Taoist Secrets of Love: Cultivating Male Sexual Energy*. New York: Aurora Press, 1984.

Clow, Barbara Hand. *Chiron: Rainbow Bridge Between the Inner and Outer Planets*. St. Paul, MN: Llewllyn Publications, 1993.

_____. *Liquid Light of Sex: Understanding Your Key Life Passages*. Santa Fe, NM: Bear & Company, 1991.

Daniélou, Alain. *Gods of Love and Ecstasy: The Traditions of Shiva and Dionysus*. Rochester, VT: Inner Traditions, 1982.

_____. *The Phallus: Sacred Symbol of Male Creative Power*. Rochester, VT: Inner Traditions, 1995.

Davies, Stevan L. *The Gospel of Thomas and Christian Wisdom.* New York: The Seabury Press, 1983.

Dee, Dr. John. *The Hieroglyphic Monad.* Boston: Weiser Books, 1975.

Diamond, Jared. *The Third Chimpanzee: The Evolution and Future of the Human Animal.* New York: HarperCollins, 1992.

Foster, Jeff. *An Extraordinary Absence: Liberation in the Midst of a Very Ordinary Life.* Salisbury, UK: Non-Duality Press, 2009.

Freke, Tim. *How Long Is Now?: A Journey to Enlightenment... and Beyond.* Carlsbad, CA: Hay House, 2009.

Friedman, David M. *A Mind of Its Own: A Cultural History of the Penis.* New York: Penguin, 2001.

Guy, David. *The Red Thread of Passion: Spirituality and the Paradox of Sex.* Boston: Shambhala, 1999.

Iyengar, B.K.S. *The Tree of Yoga.* Boston: Shambhala, 1988.

James, Geoffrey. *The Enochian Magick of Dr. John Dee: The Most Powerful System of Magick in Its Original Unexpurgated Form.* St. Paul, MN: Llewellyn, 1984, 1994.

Johns, Catherine. *Sex or Symbol: Erotic Images of Greece and Rome.* Austin, TX: University of Texas Press, 1982.

Johnson, Toby. *Gay Perspective: Things Our Homosexuality Tells Us About the Nature of God and the Universe.* Los Angeles: Alyson Books, 2003.

_____. Gay Spirituality: *The Role of Gay Identity in the Transformation of Human Consciousness.* Los Angeles: Alyson Books, 2000.

Jones, Steve. *Y: The Descent of Men.* New York: Houghton Mifflin, 2003.

Keuls, Eva C. *The Reign of the Phallus: Sexual Politics in Ancient Athens.* Berkeley: University of California Press, 1985.

Kryder, Rowena Pattee. *Foundations of Co-Creation: Alchemical Practices for Self-Realization.* Dripping Springs, TX: Golden Point Productions, 2007.

_____. *Source: Visionary Interpretations of Global Creation Myths.* Crestone, CO: Golden Point Productions, 2000.

Lanza, Robert, with Bob Berman. *Biocentrism: How Life and Consciousness are the Keys to Understanding the True Nature of the Universe.* Dallas, TX: Benbella Books, 2009.

Laqueur, Thomas W. *Solitary Sex: A Cultural History of Masturbation.* New York: Zone Books, 2003.

Leary, Timothy, Ralph Metzner, Richard Alpert. *The Psychedelic Experience: A Manual Based on the Tibetan Book of the Dead.* New York: Citadel Press, 1964, 1992.

_____. *Exo-Psychology: A Manual on the Use of the Human Nervous System According to the Instructions of the Manufacturers.* Los Angeles: Starseed/Peace Press, 1977.

_____. *Psychedelic Prayers after the Tao The Ching.* New Hyde Park, NY: University Books, 1966.

_____. *The Game of Life.* Tempe, AZ: New Falcon Publications, 1979.

Lipton, Bruce H., and Steve Bhaerman. *Spontaneous Evolution: Our Positive Future (and a Way to Get There).* Carlsbad, CA: Hay House, 2009.

Liu, Hua-Yang, Trans. Eva Wong. *Cultivating the Energy of Life.* Boston: Shambhala, 1998.

Mann, Nicholas R. His Story: *Masculinity in the Post-Patriarchal World.* St. Paul, MN: Llewellyn, 1995.

Meskell, Lynn. *Private Life in the New Kingdom.* Princeton, NJ: Princeton University Press, 2002.

Meyer, Marvin, Trans. *The Gospel of Thomas: The Hidden Sayings of Jesus.* New York: HarperSanFrancisco, 1992.

Monick, Eugene. *Phallos: Sacred Image of the Masculine.* Toronto, Canada: Inner City Books, 1987.

Morin, Jack. *Men Loving Themselves: Images of Male Self-Sexuality.* Burlingame, CA: Down There Press, 1980, 1988.

Morowitz, Harold J. *The Emergence of Everything: How the World Became Complex.* New York: Oxford University Press, 2002.

Narby, Jeremy. *Intelligence in Nature: An Inquiry into Knowledge.* New York: Jeremy P. Tarcher/Penguin, 2005.

_____. *The Cosmic Serpent: DNA and the Origins of Knowledge.* New York: Jeremy P. Tarcher/Putnam, 1998.

Naydler, Jeremy. *Shamanic Wisdom in the Pyramid Texts: The Mystical Tradition of Ancient Egypt.* Rochester, VT: Inner Traditions, 2005.

Parker, W.H. Trans. and Ed. *Priapea: Poems for a Phallic God.* New York: Croom Helm, 1988.

Rampuri. *Autobiography of a Sadhu: A Journey into Mystic India.* Rochester, VT: Destiny Books, 2005, 2010.

Reinhart, Melanie. *Chiron and the Healing Journey: An Astrological and Psychological Perspective.* Harmonsworth, UK: Penguin, 1989.

Richardson, Alan. *Earth God Rising: The Return of the Male Mysteries.* St. Paul, MN: Llewellyn, 1990.

Roscoe, Will. *Jesus and the Shamanic Tradition of Same-Sex Love.* San Francisco: Suspect Thoughts Press, 2004.

Ryan, Christopher, and Cacilda Jetha. *Sex at Dawn: The Prehistoric Origins of Modern Sexuality.* New York: Harper Collins, 2010.

Schueler, Gerald and Betty. *Enochian Magic: A practical Manual.* St. Paul, MN: Llewellyn, 1984.

Schwaller de Lubicz, R.A. *Symbol and the Symbolic: Ancient Egypt, Science, and the Evolution of Consciousness.* New York: Inner Traditions International, 1978.

_____. *The Egyptian Miracle: An Introduction to the Wisdom of the Temple.* New York: Inner Traditions International, 1985.

Schwartz, Jeffrey M., and Sharon Begley. *The Mind and the Brain: Neuroplasticity and the Power of Mental Force.* New York: ReganBooks, 2002.

St. Rain, Tedd, Introduction (ascribed to the author of Phallicism). *Nature Worship: An Account of Phallic Faiths and Practices Ancient and Modern.* Escondido, CA: The Book Tree, 1999.

Stamets, Paul. *Mycelium Running: How Mushrooms Can Help Save the World.* Berkeley: Ten Speed Press, 2005.

Tannahill, Reay. *Sex in History.* New York: A Scarborough Book, 1980.

Taylor, Timothy. *The Prehistory of Sex: Four Million Years of Human Sexual Culture.* New York: Bantam Books, 1996.

VandenBroek, André. *Al-kemi: Hermetic, Occult, Political and Private Aspects of R.A. Schwaller de Lubicz.* Great Barrington, MA: Inner Traditions/Lindisfarne Press, 1987.

Vanita, Ruth, and Saleem Kidwai, Ed. *Same-Sex Love in India: Readings from Literature and History.* New York: Palgrave, 2001.

West, John Anthony. *Serpent in the Sky: The High Wisdom of Ancient Egypt.* New York: Julian Press, 1979, 1987.

Wilson, Robert Anton. *Cosmic Trigger: The Final Secret of the Illuminati.* Tempe, AZ: New Falcon Publications, 1977.

_____. *The Illuminati Papers.* Berkeley: And/Or Press, 1980.

About the Author

Bruce P. Grether grew up in Southeast Asia. He lived in Berkeley, California off and on through the 1960s. After completion of his university studies at CSU in Colorado, Joseph Kramer's video *Fire on the Mountain* inspired his personal breakthrough in the solo cultivation of erotic energy. He learned how to transform something most men love anyway, masturbation, into a far more intense and profound experience. More information can be found at www.mm4m.org.

A Call and Invitation

to Engage in Subversive Activism

to Promote Phallic Brotherhood:

The Phallic Brotherhood Logo distills all the significance of *The Secret of the Golden Phallus* into one potent image.

Just as members of the early church used to inscribe a fish as a secret sign in order to connect with others of their faith, you can display and distribute the Phallic Brotherhood Logo to encourage and engage fellow men on the subject. *Every time the Logo is shown or seen helps to evolve the planet!* This sign for the New Millennium can be distributed simply to plants seeds of awareness. Or it may also be displayed as an invitation to other men who might wish to actually share Phallic Brotherhood with you, or who may simply wish to know more about what the Logo means.

Subvert the oppressive attitudes about the penis and masturbation!

In order to obtain stickers, shirts, ball caps and other forms of the Logo, go to: http://www.cafepress.com/brotherhoodlogo .

For more information on Mindful Masturbation and the Male Mystery School, go to:

http://www.mm4m.org/

and http://malemysteryschool.org/

or contact the author at mm4m@austin.rr.com .

Enjoy!

CPSIA information can be obtained at www.ICGtesting.com
Printed in the USA
LVOW060326160312

273211LV00003B/2/P